ATLAS OF DISEASES OF
THE ORAL MUCOSA

ATLAS OF DISEASES OF
THE ORAL MUCOSA

J. J. PINDBORG

Dental Department · University Hospital (Rigshospitalet)
Department of Oral Pathology · Royal Dental College, Copenhagen

Fourth, thoroughly revised edition

MUNKSGAARD · COPENHAGEN
North and South America:
W. B. SAUNDERS COMPANY
PHILADELPHIA · LONDON · TORONTO

ATLAS OF DISEASES OF THE ORAL MUCOSA
has been designed by the author in
collaboration with Munksgaard,
International Publishers.

Printed in Denmark by Rosendahls Bogtrykkeri, Esbjerg
Reproductions by Odense Reproduktion II, Odense
Composition by P. J. Schmidt A/S, Vojens
Cover by Lars Thorsen

ISBN 87-16-09880-3

Distributed in North and South America by
W. B. Saunders Company, Philadelphia, Pennsylvania
ISBN 0-7216-1952-5

Library of Congress catalog card No. 85-62043

Dedicated to
those who made
this atlas possible

CONTENTS

NEOPLASMS

9

ENDOCRINE, NUTRITIONAL, AND METABOLIC
DISEASES

DISEASES OF THE DIGESTIVE SYSTEM

14

COMPLICATIONS OF PREGNANCY, CHILDBIRTH AND THE PUERPERIUM

OTHER COMPLICATIONS OF PREGNANCY

DISEASES OF THE SKIN AND SUBCUTANEOUS TISSUE

LOCAL INFECTIONS OF SKIN AND SUBCUTANEOUS TISSUE

OTHER INFLAMMATORY CONDITIONS OF SKIN AND SUBCUTANEOUS TISSUE

SYMPTOMS, SIGNS AND ILL-DEFINED CONDITIONS
SYMPTOMS

INJURY AND POISONING
INJURY TO BLOOD VESSELS

BURNS

POISONING BY ANTIBIOTICS

POISONING BY OTHER ANTI-INFECTIVES

POISONING BY PRIMARILY SYSTEMATIC AGENTS

POISONING BY ANALGESICS, ANTIPYRETICS AND
ANTIRHEUMATICS

POISONING BY ANTICONVULSANTS

18

PREFACE

In this fourth edition of the Atlas, the text has been thoroughly revised and updated, no fewer than 26 new diseases have been added to the present edition, and 225 new references have been included in the bibliography. As before, the basic principle followed in preparing the bibliography has been to select recent papers giving the most comprehensive discussion of the oral aspects of the diseases in question.

The main emphasis has been placed on the clinical diagnostic aspects of the diseases; histopathology has been dealt with only when necessary for the understanding of a given disease.

The author is fully aware that some diseases are still lacking, but is confident that future editions will be able to fill some of the gaps.

As in the previous editions the classification of the diseases of the oral mucosa is based upon the "Application of the International Classification of Diseases to dentistry and stomatology" (second edition) published by the World Health Organization in 1978. At the end of the Atlas, the code numbers are provided for all the diseases discussed.

The material for this Atlas has been collected mainly in the Dental Department of the University Hospital (Rigshospitalet) in Copenhagen, and the majority of the patients have been photographed with a Hasselblad camera. The author expresses his appreciation of the skillful work by the Department's photographer. He is also grateful to all dentists and physicians who have referred patients through the years.

January 1985

Jens J. Pindborg

Atlas

Tuberculosis

Tuberculous involvement of the oral mucosa is rarely seen. Its frequency of occurrence varies, according to the literature, from 0.05 to 1.4 percent[403]. Most rare is an oral manifestation of primary tuberculosis. When an oral tuberculous ulcer is observed, it is most often secondary to far advanced pulmonary tuberculosis[375]. There has been some discussion as to the origin of such lesions. As the oral mucosa obviously possesses a high resistance to invasion by the tubercle bacillus, it seems most probable that the tuberculous oral mucosal lesion is the result of a hematogenous spread of bacilli from a focus elsewhere in the body. The most frequent seat of an oral tuberculous ulceration is the dorsum of the tongue, followed by the lips. Usually, the oral tuberculous lesion is an ulceration with an irregular outline and undermined borders, covered by a yellowish-grayish fibrinous layer. At the mucocutaneous junction, the ulcer is characteristically shallow with a granulating base[560]. The patient shown here is a 40-year-old woman who suffers from pulmonary tuberculosis. The ulceration has not caused any pain, and it was detected incidentally. A biopsy and a culture are necessary to make the diagnosis. (Courtesy of Dr. A. JEPSEN, Aarhus, Denmark).

Atypical tuberculosis

Although the typical tuberculous lesion of the oral mucosa is an irregular ulceration with ragged, undermined edges surrounded by a red zone, the clinical features may occasionally be of a different type. Such a manifestation, located on the palate, is illustrated in the picture which is of a 41-year-old woman. The painless lesion, which was incidentally diagnosed at a routine dental check-up, is slightly elevated and nodular with a spotty, dark reddish color. A biopsy showed numerous granulomas composed of epithelial cells, multinucleated giant cells of the Langhans type, and a lymphocytic infiltration, but acid-fast bacilli could not be demonstrated. At the age of 25 years the patient contracted pulmonary tuberculosis and lupus vulgaris capitis. She received treatment with PAS, isoniazid, and streptomycin and since the age of 30 her pulmonary infection had been under control. After the palatal biopsy, a thorough examination failed to reveal any active foci of tuberculosis. Five months after the biopsy, the patient developed an eczema affecting the entire body which was diagnosed as tuberculosis cutis lichenoides. The unusual case has been explained as a hyperergic sensitivity to tuberculin.

24

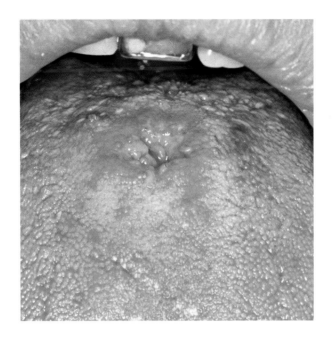

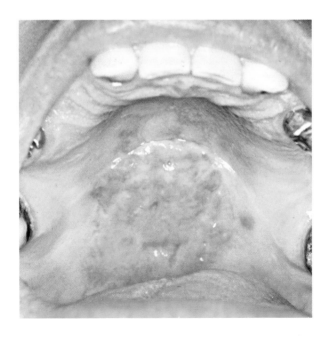

Leprosy

Leprosy is restricted mainly to tropical and subtropical countries. According to WHO estimates, there are still approximately ten million lepers, mainly in Africa, Japan, South America, and Southeast Asia. Leprosy is a chronic, insidious, contagious, granulomatous disease, which is caused by *Mycobacterium leprae* and has a long incubation period, sometimes of many years' duration. Leprosy may assume several clinical forms. Roughly, the two major types are *tuberculoid* leprosy and *lepromatous* leprosy. Whereas the main feature of the tuberculoid type is macular lesions on the skin, the lepromatous type is characterized by infiltrates in the deeper corium and the deeper cutaneous layers which form nodular masses, lepromas. Although nodules may develop on any part of the body, the face is often the first area involved. The illustration of a patient from Kerala in South India shows a nodular infiltrate on the right buccal mucosa and commissure. Lepromatous oral lesions, which are found in 20 percent of the patients with lepromatous leprosy, also may occur in the soft palate[458], on the dorsum of the tongue, the lips, and the lingual gingiva[329]. (Courtesy of the late Dr. J. ZACHARIAH, Trivandrum, India).

Streptococcal gingivostomatitis

Gingivitis or gingivostomatitis caused by streptococci exists, although it is rarely described in the literature[66]. The disease usually is preceded by an attack of tonsillitis[334], and the gingiva becomes diffusely and acutely inflamed, red, and swollen, with an increased tendency to bleed. Occasionally gingival abscesses are present in the interdental papillae. The submandibular lymph nodes are enlarged and tender. Previously, *Streptococcus viridans* was considered to be the causative organism. Recent evidence associates the infection with β-hemolytic streptococci. The picture illustrates the gingival appearance in a 20-year-old woman. Two days before onset of oral signs, the patient had a sore throat and an elevated temperature. The entire gingiva is affected, being fiery red and swollen. In some areas the gingiva is the site of discrete, yellowish elements, which can be scraped off, leaving a bleeding surface. In various parts of the oral mucosa, especially the lips, similar lesions are found. Cultures from the lesions yielded hemolytic streptococci of group F. In contrast to acute necrotizing gingivitis, streptococcal gingivostomatitis does not lead to a loss of gingival tissue.

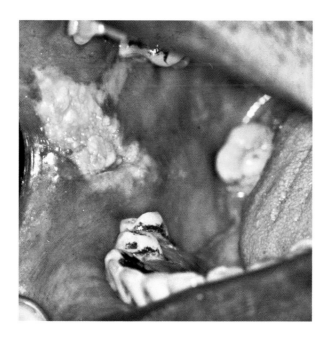

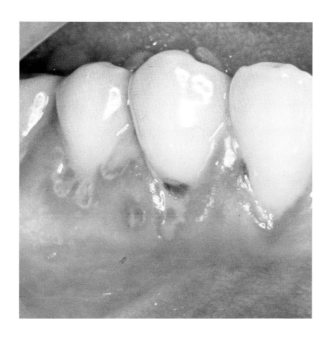

Scarlatina

Scarlatina, scarlet fever, is an acute contagious disease caused by group A streptococci which produce an erythrogenic toxin giving rise to a characteristic skin rash. After an incubation period of 2 to 4 days the disease begins with chills, vomiting and sore throat followed by increased temperature and rapid pulse. The diffuse bright scarlet erythema usually appears on the second day of the disease with a variable distribution. The face, especially the temples and the cheeks, is flushed and red, but a pale area, the circumoral pallor is often seen around the mouth. The oral mucosa appears red and swollen, especially the buccal and labial mucosa. In the palate there may be a punctate redness. About the second to fifth day, small milk-white patches may be seen on the buccal mucosa representing desquamated epithelium. The most characteristic oral manifestation of scarlatina is found on the tongue which early in the course of the infection is heavily coated and grayish. Soon the tongue becomes fiery red with large fungiform papillae (raspberry tongue). By the fourth to fifth day there is complete lingual desquamation with multiple papillary elevations which are sometimes called "strawberry tongue". This change is seen on the tongue of the 10-year-old girl pictured opposite.

Actinomycosis

Actinomycosis is a chronic suppurative and granulomatous disease caused by *Actinomyces Israëli*. Most often actinomycosis is localized in the cervicofacial region. It is most prevalent between 15 and 35 years of age, and is found twice as often in men as in women. The cervicofacial actinomycosis usually is localized in the submandibular area or around the angle of the jaw in the form of an elevated, very firm swelling, which is frequently red or purplish. Sometimes trismus may be present. The *Actinomyces Israëli* gain entrance into the soft tissues through open necrotic pulps, radicular cysts, wounds[473], or impacted teeth. The woody and chronic nature of the lesion may raise suspicion of a malignant tumor. As the lesion grows, multiple abscesses develop, breaking through the skin in several areas and causing a characteristic pattern of multiple sinus. Out of these may come the so-called sulfur granules which represent colonies of actinomycetes. The diagnosis depends almost entirely on the bacteriologic examination of the discharge. Actinomycosis localized in the oral mucosa is quite rare. Several cases affecting the tongue have been reported[143], and the illustration shows an actinomycotic process in the buccal mucosa of a 20-year-old man.

28

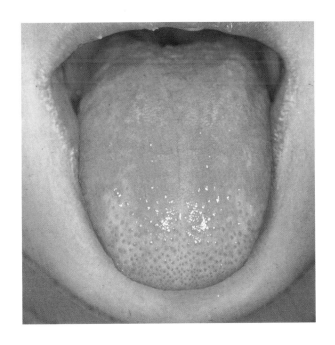

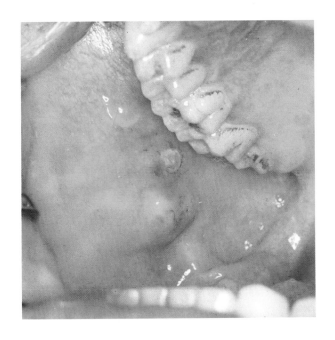

Chickenpox

Chickenpox (varicella) and herpes zoster are different clinical manifestations of infection with the same virus[67], *herpesvirus varicellae*. Chickenpox apparently results from contact of the nonimmune host with virus, whereas herpes zoster is thought to be infection in a particularly immune host. Chickenpox is a generalized, highly contagious disease, principally affecting children. Following an incubation period of 10 to 20 days, a vesicular eruption appears on the skin, profusely over the thorax, proximal extremities and scalp. The skin of the hand is not affected. The rash, which begins abruptly, consists of discrete erythematous, maculopapular lesions in which vesiculation quickly takes place. According to some authors intraoral manifestations occur in most patients, the mucosal lesions frequently preceding cutaneous involvement. All areas of the oral mucosa may be affected[33], most often in the form of discrete yellow-colored vesicles which quickly become ulcerated[177]. The illustration shows palatal lesions in an 11-year-old boy. The painless lesions are ulcerated and surrounded by a distinct red halo. The rest of the oral mucosa, larynx, and the eyes are rarely involved. (Courtesy of Dr. M. ESPELID, Bergen, Norway).

Herpes zoster

Herpes zoster (shingles) most probably is caused by reactivation of varicella virus lying dormant in sensory ganglia of patients whose immunity to the virus has diminished. Herpes zoster has a tendency of increasing in incidence with age and approximately 20 percent of reported cases involve the trigeminal nerve[266]. When the second or third divisions of the trigeminal nerve are affected, oral manifestations may occur in addition to the skin lesions. Pain and an itching sensation precede both skin and mucosal lesions. The skin affections usually appear before the oral manifestation. The latter consists of groups of unilaterally occurring vesicles surrounded by a distinct erythematous zone affecting any part of the oral mucosa. Vesicles are clearly seen on the gingiva and labial mucosa of the 25-year-old man shown here. He was referred for uncharacteristic pain in the right side of the mouth, where no clinical changes of the mucosa could be observed. Two days later oral vesicles developed together with a conjunctivitis of the right eye. On clinical grounds, the unilateral location of the vesicles, a diagnosis of herpes zoster was made. Owing to the humid environment in the oral cavity and frequent exposure to trauma, the vesicles will soon burst and coalesce, leaving erosions.

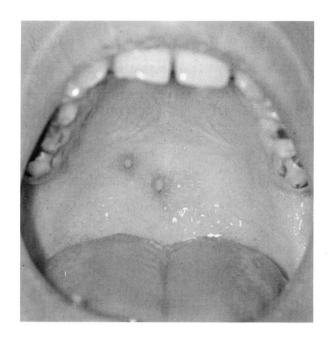

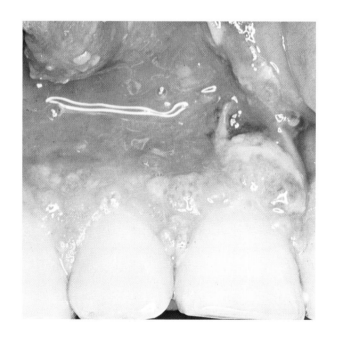

Herpes zoster

The unilateral pattern of a herpes zoster infection is obvious in the illustrated case of a 70-year-old man with a herpes zoster infection of the
trigeminal nerve. The left side of the tongue is the seat of fibrin-covered
ulcerations which are in the process of healing. The patient also had
lesions on the left buccal mucosa and palate. The most frequently affected
areas of the oral mucosa are the lips, tongue, hard and soft palate, and
buccal mucosa[264]. The pain associated with the oral lesions is quite severe.
Occasionally the pain may simulate a pulpitis. The incidence of herpes
zoster is increased in patients with a low general resistance and in patients
receiving corticosteroids or cytostatic/immunosuppressive drugs[576] or having a systemic malignancy. The oral manifestations may then develop in
a rather dramatic way ending in loss of teeth, osteomyelitis, and extensive
necrosis of the jaw bone with sequestration[609]. So far, no satisfactory
explanation has been given for the mechanism by which herpes zoster
induces necrosis of the jaws. Patients with Hodgkin's disease have a very
high risk of developing a herpes zoster infection. Few cases of an intraoral
herpes zoster affection without skin lesions have been reported[158].

Herpes labialis

Herpes labialis, also known as "fever blister" or "cold sore", is caused by
the *Herpesvirus hominis* Type 1 (HSV-1)[247] and is characterized by a
vesicular eruption on the skin adjacent to or on the vermilion border
itself. In an unselected Swedish population sample[24] herpes labialis was
found in 3 percent. If those who had had an attack at least once during
the previous 2 years were included the prevalence rose to 17 percent. The
majority of the adult population has sustained herpetic infection, although
it may not have become clinically manifest. The herpes simplex virus may
be "dormant" in a particular area, and vesicles may appear when the
patient becomes exposed to sunlight, to a febrile disease, or occasionally
in relation to menstruation[590]. Herpes labialis is preceded by an itching
in the affected area. Within 12 hours vesicles develop and the vesicles
rupture to form ulcers and crusts in 36 to 48 hours. Most patients loose
the crust and have healed lesions by day 8 to 10[406]. Fever and lymphadenopathy may also appear before the vesicles. The patient shown here is a
24-year-old woman suffering from an eruption of herpes labialis after a
common cold. In the U.S.A. there is a decrease in the prevalence and
severity of recurrent herpes labialis since 1958[515].

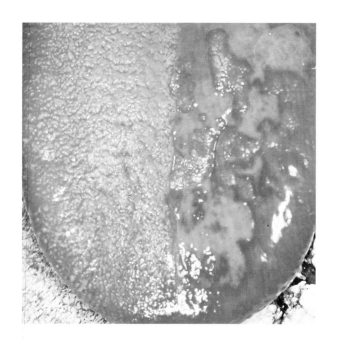

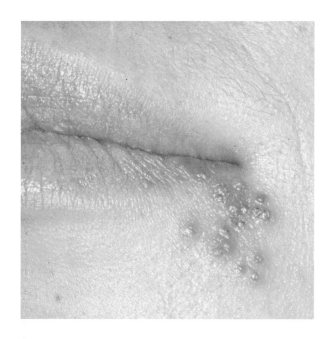

Herpetic gingivostomatitis

When the herpes simplex virus affects the oral mucosa it results in a herpetic gingivostomatitis, often erroneously diagnosed as an acute necrotizing gingivitis. The herpetic gingivostomatitis, however, is not, like the acute necrotizing gingivitis, associated with destruction of the gingiva. Herpetic gingivostomatitis, a rather common disease, is usually seen in children between the ages of 2 and 4 years. The incubation period is about 1 week. The disease is characterized by a sudden development of fever, general malaise, regional lymphadenopathy, and oral lesions consisting of a marked acute gingivitis and small vesicles occurring in the oral mucosa. The painful gingivitis, which affects the marginal as well as the attached gingiva, is characterized by fiery red, swollen gingiva. Often the marginal gingiva is covered by a serofibrinous exudate. The picture illustrates a typical case in a 2-year-old girl where a number of burst vesicles are present on the labial mucosa. Sometimes the elements on the vermilion border will cause formation of crust. The oral lesions will usually heal in 10 to 14 days. In a number of cases nail infections are the result of auto-inoculation of virus by nail-biting. Some adenoviruses occasionally produce lesions of the palate that are indistinguishable from those caused by herpes simplex virus[290].

Herpetic gingivostomatitis

Epidemics of herpetic gingivostomatitis have been reported in several countries; some have occurred in institutions. Most of the epidemics are of a mild nature, although outbreaks have been described with a surprisingly high death rate, owing to the development of encephalitis[232]. In a number of such cases autopsy has revealed a generalized herpes simplex infection. A more severe course of herpetic infection usually can be expected when the affected population is malnourished. In some developing countries the prevalence of herpetic gingivostomatitis is quite high, and often is associated with a superimposed acute necrotizing gingivitis[163]. The disease is by no means confined only to 2- to 4-year-old children. The picture illustrates palatal lesions in a 51-year-old man with herpetic gingivostomatitis. A sample of 164 cases among adults had a mean age of 32 years. In most cases the herpetic gingivostomatitis will not recur, but some patients have been reported with an intraoral recurrent form of herpes simplex virus infection with the lesions occurring most commonly on gingiva and hard palate[587]. Exfoliative cytology has been found to reveal cellular changes with specific virus-induced nuclear alterations[519].

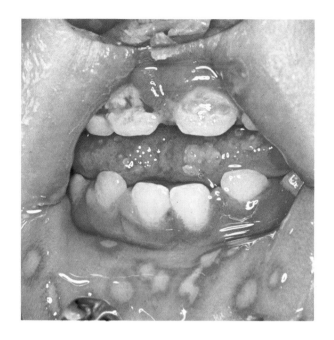

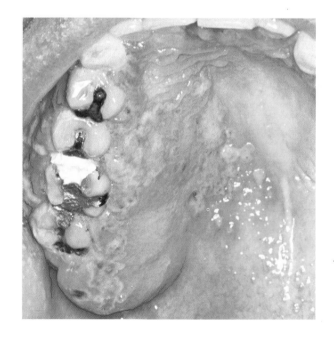

Measles

One of the most common exanthematous childhood diseases is measles (in "English" Latin called rubeola, and in "German" Latin morbilli) caused by a filtrate virus. After an incubation period of 2 weeks, this highly contagious disease begins with chills, fever, coryza, cough, and conjunctivitis. Then appear the Koplik's spots on the oral, genital and eye mucosa[543]. Three days after the initial fever, a dusky-red, papular skin eruption appears. The rash is first seen behind the ears and on the forehead, and then spreads to the entire body. The oral manifestations of measles consist of: (1) a nonspecific stomatitis characterized by a diffuse erythema, mainly affecting the palate and pharynx; (2) the appearance of Koplik's spots on the buccal mucosa. These lesions are small, irregular, bluish-white spots on an erythematous base. The spots, which may occur also on the inside of the lips, vary in number. Occasionally, although they may cover the entire buccal mucosa, as in the 6-year-old boy opposite, the more usual site is the occlusal line. The spots fade as the skin rash appears. In tropical countries measles may be complicated by cancrum oris (p. 178). (Courtesy of Dr. H. P. PHILIPSEN, Aarhus, Denmark).

Herpangina

Herpangina, caused by strains of Coxsackie virus group A type 4, was described in 1920[616]. It is a mild disease, occurring most often during the summer and early autumn. Although it occasionally occurs in adults, as in the case of the 23-year-old man shown here, the highest incidence is found in infants and young children. Spread is from person to person with an incubation period of about 4 days (2–9 days), after which the patients experience an elevated temperature, general malaise, vomiting, abdominal pain, headache and muscle pain. Vesicles appear on the anterior pillars of the tonsillar fauces, the soft palate, the uvula, and the tonsils. The vesicles are of pinhead size, surrounded by a halo, and gradually progress to slightly larger ulcers covered by fibrin. The lesions last for only 3–5 days, and then heal quickly. The most important differential diagnosis to be considered is acute herpetic gingivostomatitis, from which herpangina can be distinguished by the fact that acute gingivitis is not present in herpangina. Furthermore, herpetic gingivostomatitis is characterized by longer duration and more severe pain. Herpangina is selflimiting, and the prognosis is excellent.

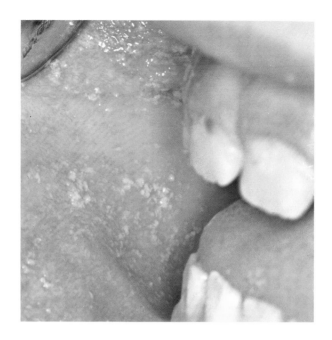

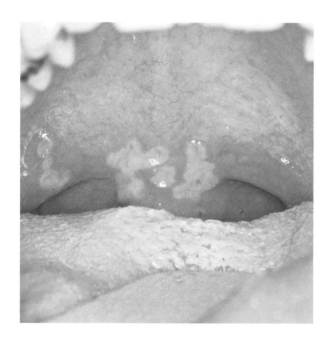

Vesicular stomatitis with exanthem

Epidemics of this disease, also called "hand-foot-mouth disease", have been reported in several countries[252]. This mild infection is caused by a Coxsackie virus, group A 16 (sometimes A 5 and A 10 or group B 2 and 5)[331] with an incubation time of 1–7 days. In an epidemic affecting 742 persons in Singapore, the morbidity rate was highest in children under 5 years of age[210]. The disease, which usually lasts a week, occasionally is accompanied by a low grade fever. The skin lesions consist of painless vesicles occurring on the hands and feet, and of a maculopapular rash on the buttocks. The vesicles, sometimes preceded by a red macula, are found most often on the buccal mucosa, but also on the mucosal part of lips, palate, tongue, and the gingiva as in the 26-year-old man shown here. The vesicles, ranging in size from 1 to 10 mm in diameter, will burst, leaving a grayish-yellow ulcer with surrounding erythema. An outbreak of the disease among students and staff members of a dental school has been described[103] and transmission of the infection to a dentist following his examination of an already infected patient has been reported[529]. In Japan there have been epidemics of hand-foot-and-mouth disease caused by enterovirus 71 with central nervous system disorders in 8 to 24 percent leading to death in some cases[271].

Infectious mononucleosis

Infectious mononucleosis is an acute and usually benign infectious disease characterized by fever, angina, enlarged lymph nodes, presence of atypical lymphocytes, and the appearance of heterophile antibody in the blood, and is caused by the Epstein-Barr virus. Usually, infectious mononucleosis is a disease of young adults. After an incubation period of 5 to 15 days, the disease may have either an abrupt or a gradual onset, and will most often run a course of 1 month. The most consistent sign is lymphadeno pathy, with the posterior cervical lymph nodes invariably involved. Lesions in the oral cavity are often the first clinical symptoms[97]. Whereas gingivo-stomatitis and gingival ulcerations may be seen, it is the occurrence of palatal petechiae which is the most conspicuous oral sign, and these were found in 41 percent in one sample of 80 patients[150]. The petechiae appear as sharply circumscribed red spots, about 0.5 mm to 1 mm in diameter. Located at the junction of the hard and soft palates, the petechiae may occur either in groups or singly, as in the 19-year-old man pictured op-posite. The petechiae will decrease with remission of other symptoms. (Courtesy of Dr. M. ESPELID, Bergen, Norway).

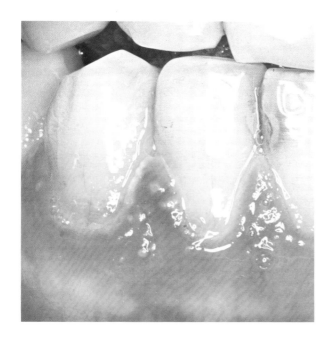

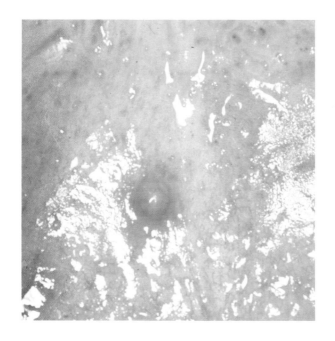

Viral wart

Also known as verrucae vulgares, warts caused by human papillomavirus (HPV) may be found in the oral mucosa[281]. The proof has been the presence of HPV antigens in the oral epithelium, where the positive reaction is found intranuclear in cells in the superficial epithelium[281]. The majority of oral warts are seen in children who also have warts on their fingers. When the child chews on the warts, the virus is transmitted to the oral mucosa. Previously, the oral mucosa was considered an unusual site for warts, but more recently it has been stated that the incidence of involvement of the oral mucosa has become substantial[361]. Viral warts may be located any place in the oral mucosa, although the lips and tongue are the preferred sites, probably because they are most exposed during the chewing of finger warts. The picture illustrates a number of viral warts in a 60-year-old man who had several warts on his fingers and admitted to chewing on the warts. The viral warts usually are flat and whitish, with a papillomatous surface, although pedunculated lesions may be seen. They appear suddenly, and their growth is quite rapid. Clinically, verrucae vulgares cannot be distinguished from papillomas (p. 100).

Condyloma acuminatum

Condyloma acuminatum is a papillomatous growth which occurs most frequently on anogenital skin and mucosa but may also involve other warm, moist, intertriginous areas. Condyloma acuminatum is a quite common venereal disease today. The etiologic agent has been established as a papilloma virus of the papova group. Since it was demonstrated that inoculation of a bacteria-free and cell-free extract of condyloma acuminatum into human skin produces verruca vulgaris or verruca plana, and inoculation into mucous membrane produces condylomata, it is generally believed that condyloma acuminatum and verruca vulgaris are lesions caused by identical viruses, but showing different clinical and pathologic manifestations according to the site where they attack[440]. Condylomas start as multiple, small, pink nodules which often proliferate and coalesce to form soft, sessile, or pedunculated papillary growths. Oral manifestations are rare, judging from the very few reports in the literature. The picture shows a condyloma of the lateral border of the tongue of a 32-year-old man who also had a similar lesion sublingually. The wife of the patient had genital condylomas and the transmission is supposed to have been through orogenital contact.

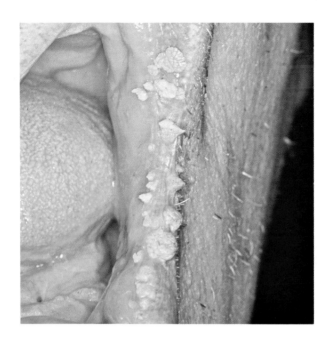

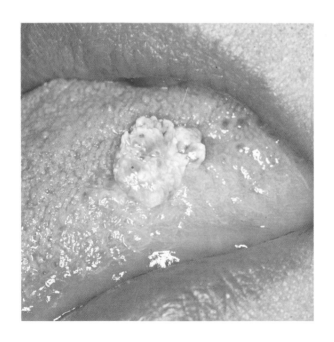

Condyloma acuminatum

Oral condylomas have a more cauliflower- than papillomatous-like surface, as is obvious in the illustration on p. 39. The disease may appear also as small lesions with a verruca vulgaris-like morphology. A condyloma may present itself as an epulis, i.e. a growth originating from the gingiva. This location is shown in the picture opposite, which is of a 28-year-old man. Two months before admission, condylomas were diagnosed around the anus and on the penis. Basically, the sessile gingival lesion presents the same morphologic features as the lesion of the tongue illustrated on p. 41. The wife of the patient had been treated for vaginal condylomas, and also in this case an orogenital contact was the likely mode of transmission, as has also been demonstrated by other investigators[352]. The transmission may also occur from perianal lesions[542]. Oral condylomas tend to recur, as has been shown in a patient with extensive gingival condylomas[500]. One of the reasons for the very few reports on oral condylomas is probably that they have been diagnosed as papillomas, verrucae, or fibroepithelial papillomas. In contrast to papillomas and verrucae, oral condylomas are characterized by a slight parakeratosis or even an unkeratinized surface.

Leishmaniasis

Leishmaniasis is an infection with a protozoan parasite of the genus *Leishmania*. It is transmitted by the bite of sandflies (Phlebotomus). There are several species, of which some have oral manifestations. Only the mucocutaneous South American form (epundia), caused by *Leishmania Braziliensis*, will be dealt with here. In some areas 10 to 20 percent of the population are infected. After an incubation period varying from a few days to several months, the intitial skin lesion, usually on the legs but often on the face, enlarges progressively. Dissemination follows either by direct extension or by lymphatics to the mouth, pharynx, and nose. There may be an interval of many years between the primary and mucocutaneous lesions. In the nose, destruction of the nasal septum and oropharynx occurs, and death may result from secondary infection of the respiratory passages. In the mouth the hard palate may be destroyed. The illustration shows a palatal lesion in a Venezuelan with a granulomatous pattern. The diagnosis is made by observation of the lesion clinically and biopsy, skin reaction, the Montenegro test, cytologic smears and appropriate cultures[96]. (Courtesy of Dr. R. A. LOBO, Caracas, Venezuela).

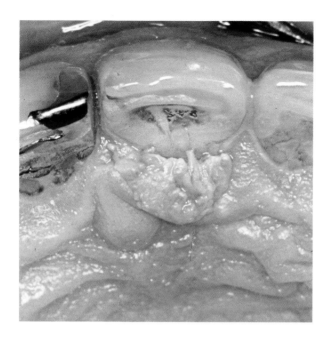

RICKETTSIOSES AND OTHER ARTHROPOD-BORNE DISEASES

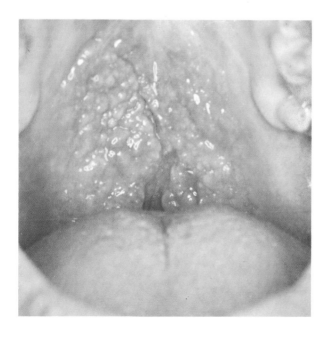

Circumoral furrows in congenital syphilis

A characteristic late effect of congenital syphilis is illustrated opposite. This is a 47-year-old woman who sought dental advice for an angular cheilosis, which she thought was caused by a new set of dentures. A clinical and serologic examination showed that she suffered from congenital syphilis. The circumoral furrows (also called syphilitic rhagades or Parrot's furrows) due to congenital syphilis are the result of a diffuse syphilitic infiltrative process in this area from the third to the seventh week of life. Today, earlier diagnosis and use of antibiotics limit the amount of scarring. Thus, a review from 1970 of 217 patients with late congenital syphilis showed only 8 percent with syphilitic rhagades[191]. The furrows are not true scars, but are due to an atrophy of the elastic tissue in the corium[537]. The scars resemble the spokes of a wheel, radiating from the angles of the eyes, nose, mouth, chin[191]. Areas of greater mobility, such as the lower lip, are said to be more prone to the formation of furrows. The movements cause epithelial ruptures perpendicular to the mucocutaneous border as well as to the underlying muscles. In contrast to the changes caused by ill-fitting dentures, syphilitic furrows extend into the vermilion border, which shows a decreased intensity of color and an indistinct border toward the skin.

Primary syphilis

Syphilis is capable of producing a large variety of manifestations in the oral mucosa. After an incubation period of 3 to 5 weeks, the primary lesion, the chancre, develops. The primary lesion usually is accompanied by swollen, painless, regional lymph nodes. Of all chancres, 5 to 10 percent are extragenital; half of these are located on the oral mucosa. A recent French study[124] has shown a male:female ratio for primary syphilis to be 9:1. Among the oral manifestations, the most common site is the lower vermilion border, but other areas, including the tongue and the gingiva[535], may be affected. A palatal chancre in a 23-year-old man is illustrated opposite. Usually, the chancre is a painless, dark-reddish, elevated, ulcerated, and indurated lesion varying in size from a few millimeters to from 2 to 3 cm. The diagnosis should be made on a combination of the clinical findings, dark-field examination of smears from the lesion, and serologic reactions, but it should be remembered that the serologic reaction does not become positive until 4–5 weeks after the infection. After a period of some weeks the chancre heals spontaneously. (Courtesy of Dr. A. PERDRUP, Copenhagen, Denmark).

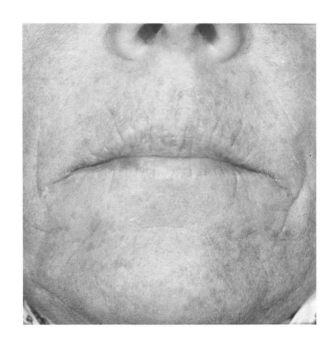

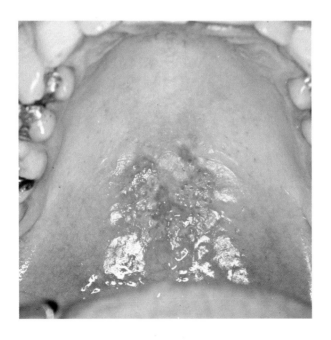

Mucous patches in secondary syphilis

Signs of secondary syphilis, in the form of cutaneous eruptions, sore throat, and general enlargement of the lymph nodes, usually appear 6 weeks after the primary stage. A longer period, up to 2 years, may also be experienced before the secondary manifestations appear. The secondary stage may begin with mild fever, headache, anorexia, and malaise. The cutaneous eruptions may take several forms: macular, papular, maculopapular, pustular, or lichenoid[311]. The sore throat is caused by swollen and inflamed tonsils; a hoarseness is often present. The generalized adenopathy consists of painless, palpable nodes. At the angles of the mouth, moist, flat papules (called condylomata lata or split paules) may appear. These papules may resemble candidosis infection, and quite often are located in this area. Another characteristic feature is the mucous patches, which are also seen in the oral mucosa. In some cases the mucous patches may be the only manifestations of the secondary stage, for which reason the diagnosis may be difficult to make[190]. The picture illustrates a 19-year-old woman in the secondary stage of syphilis. She has mucous patches on the tongue, the buccal mucosa, and the lower labial mucosa.

Mucous patches in secondary syphilis

The oral mucous patches in secondary syphilis are slightly raised, grayish-white lesions usually surrounded by a red halo. When the covering necrotic slough is scraped off, a raw, bleeding surface appears. The mucous patches may occur as solitary lesions, but usually several patches are found simultaneously in the oral mucosa. The favored site is the tongue, probably because this location is more exposed to trauma. The illustration, from a 20-year-old woman, shows the type of a syphilitic mucous patch, which resembles a snail track. On both sides of the illustrated lesion the patient had similar affections on the labial mucosa. The differential diagnosis may sometimes be difficult, especially if the lesions are dominated by an erythematous element. The following conditions may resemble syphilitic mucous patches: candidiasis, herpetic gengivostomatitis, erythema multiforme exudativum, erosive lichen planus, and leukoplakia, as in the illustrated case. The mucous patches are the most contagious lesions in acute syphilis because of their high content of spirochetes. Many cases are known of dentists and physicians who have contracted syphilis by palpating oral structures with unprotected fingers.

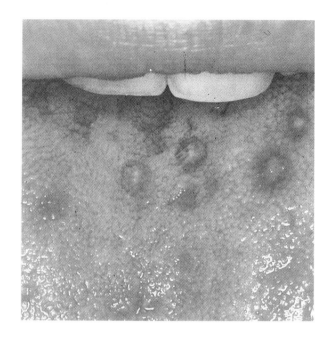

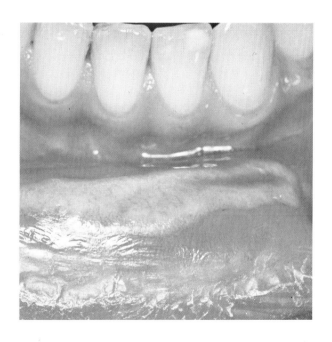

Palatal perforation in tertiary syphilis

Tertiary syphilis may give rise to a number of different oral lesions. Best known is perforation of the palate. The perforation is caused by the gumma, consisting of granulation tissue with caseous necrosis and giant cells. The gumma is a destructive lesion. It appears as a raised, firm, rubbery infiltration, which undergoes ulceration and necrosis, due to a vasculitis, leading to the denudation of underlying bone. When located in the hard palate, the end result may be a perforation into the nasal cavity. The perforations vary in size. The illustration shows an extensive destruction of the palate in a 76-year-old woman, who had been infected by syphilis 50 years before. The nasal septum can be seen, together with the conchae inferiores and mediae. The gumma may be located on the soft palate also, causing either destruction of the uvula or perforation of the mucosa, occasionally in the form of multiple holes[619]. An ulcerated gumma may be mistaken for a malignant tumor. It should be mentioned that the palate may be the site of tertiary syphilitic manifestations other than the gumma, in the form of granulomas.

Atrophic glossitis in tertiary syphilis

Tongue lesions often are seen in patients with tertiary syphilis. They comprise ulcerative glossitis, sclerotic glossitis, and gummatous glossitis[40]. Described as bald tongue or atrophic glossitis, the earliest change is a condition in which there is an atrophy of the filiform and fungiform papillae. This is brought about by a diffuse vasculitis, eventually resulting in an obliterative endarteritis with a circulatory deficiency to the lingual surface[372]. The patient shown here is a 47-year-old woman who sought dental advice because of an angular cheilosis and dryness of the oral mucosa. A clinical-serologic examination revealed tertiary syphilis, also manifesting itself by the Argyll Robertson's pupil. The pale tongue surface exhibits an almost total loss of papillae, and the middle part of the dorsum of the tongue has a slightly lobulated appearance. Furthermore, there is a bilateral angular cheilosis. The atrophic syphilitic glossitis is quite often associated with leukoplakias, which do not differ morphologically from those due solely to tobacco and other irritants, although a leukoplakia, as the one shown on p. 194, affecting the surface of the tongue should raise suspicion of a syphilitic background.

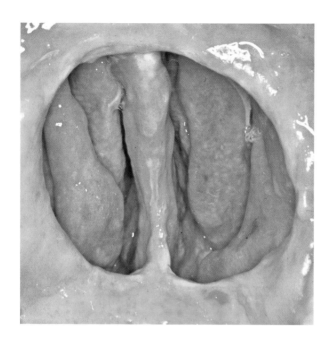

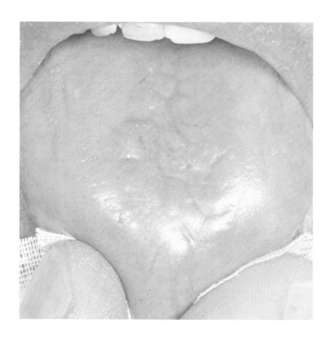

Interstitial glossitis and carcinoma in tertiary syphilis

The gumma appearing in the third stage of the syphilitic infection may occur in any part of the oral cavity, although the palate and the tongue are preferred sites. Gummatous involvement of the tongue may occur either as a solitary gumma or as multiple small gummata. A superficially located gumma may simulate a malignant tumor. The occurrence of small healing gummata causes syphilitic glossitis, leading to a lingua lobata, sometimes associated with macroglossia. The results of an interstitial syphilitic glossitis are illustrated in a 68-year-old man who was infected with syphilis 27 years before. The surface of the tongue is also the site of leukoplakic changes, and on the tip of the tongue a squamous cell carcinoma has developed. It has been found that syphilis is more common among patients with carcinoma of the anterior two-thirds of the tongue than among controls[612]. It is, however, questioned whether this correlation is due to a syphilitic glossitis or to the treatment with the arsenic compounds used before 1940. Thus, a study[371] from 1958 has indicated that the percentage of patients with both lingual carcinoma and a positive history of syphilis is not presently as high as hitherto reported.

Gonococcal stomatitis

Considering the great range of variations within sexual life, it seems surprising that primary gonorrheal infections are almost exclusively confined to the genital tract and conjunctivae and rarely seen on the oral mucosa. The illustration is from the oral cavity of a 30-year-old man in whose urethral discharge gonococci were demonstrated microscopically and by cultivation. He had previously been treated four times for uncomplicated urethral gonorrhea. On examination the patient complained of an itching and burning sensation localized in the buccal sulci and facial gingiva, and some of the interdental papillae were necrotic. Yellowish pseudomembranes, which could be scraped off, leaving a bleeding surface, covered the lesions. The oral mucosa as a whole was fiery red, and the viscosity of the saliva was increased. On questioning, the patient reported that prior to normal coitus he usually performed cunnilingus, this ceremony usually lasting for some 10 minutes. Examination of his fiancée revealed a gonococcal genital infection. After one treatment with penicillin, the oral changes as well as the urethritis disappeared within 3 days[490]. Since this case was reported in 1961 only very few similar cases have appeared in the literature[277].

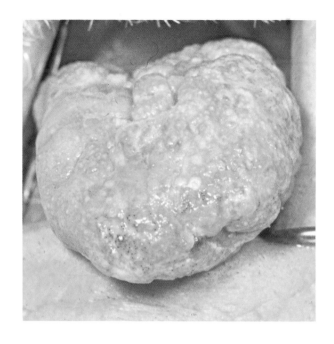

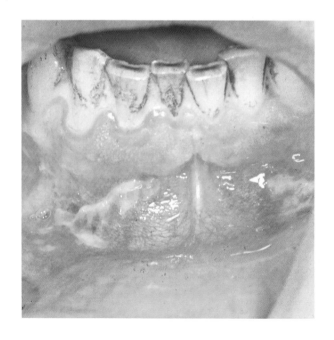

Gonococcal dermatitis syndrome

After 1971, when the first report came on gonococcal tonsillar infection[78], a number of articles have appeared on the subject[276]. There may be a superficial similarity with acute tonsillitis, pharyngeal diphtheria, pharyngeal streptococcal infection, scarlet fever, and infectious mononucleosis. When there is suspicion of a gonococcal tonsillitis, a smear should be taken and cultures performed. Oral manifestations of a gonococcal infection may also occur as part of the gonococcal dermatitis syndrome, a goncoccal sepsis characterized clinically by fever, arthritis, and dermatitis brought about by small infarctions[125]. Lesions usually present as vesiculopustules, sometimes hemorrhagic; they are few in number and show a predilection for the extremities. Gonococci are either not demonstrable or detectable for only brief periods. There is discussion on whether the gonococci in the oral lesions have been available from either an orogenital contact or from the blood stream because of a gonococcemia, but a close time relationship to the occurrence of dermatitis favors a metastatic pathogenesis[125]. The illustration is of a characteristic tongue lesion in a 50-year-old woman who also had several pustular lesions on the skin. (Courtesy of Dr. N. HJORTH, Copenhagen, Denmark)

Reiter's syndrome

The term Reiter's syndrome, previously used for the triad of arthritis, conjunctivitis, and urethritis now comprises a much wider spectrum of symptomatology. Although the etiology is still unknown, the histocompatibility antigen HLA-B 27 has been found to be present in up to 80–95 percent of the patients. The syndrome usually occurs in young men between 20 and 30 years of age. In 68 percent in a Finnish study[305] of 173 patients, urethritis, probably sexually transmitted, was the first manifestation of the disease. Joint involvement was seen in 98 percent. Penile lesions, as a circinate balanitis, are mainly limited to the foreskin and glans. The prevalence of oral manifestations shows pronounced variations in different surveys[421]; in the Finnish survey it was 17 percent. The lesions seen on the oral mucosa are usually red, slightly elevated areas, varying from 1 mm to several cm in size and sometimes surrounded by a whitish circinate line, as seen in the picture, which illustrates a lesion on the palate of a 35-year-old man with Reiter's syndrome. The oral lesions may also have the appearance of small, opaque vesicles or areas of glistening erythema exhibiting a granular surface[211].

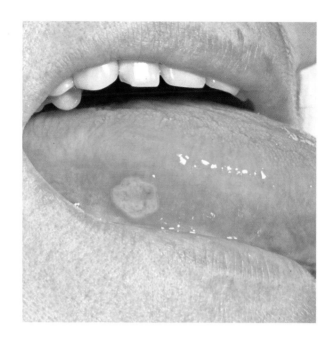

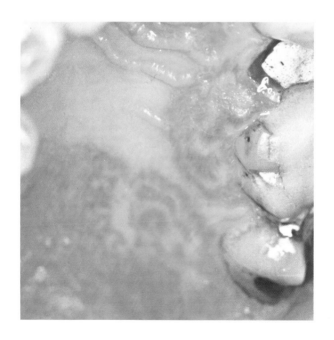

Acute necrotizing gingivitis

Acute necrotizing gingivitis (ANG) is known under many other names, the foremost being Vincent's gingivitis, but terms like "trench mouth", "ulceromembranous gingivitis", and "acute necrotic ulcerative gingivitis" also are frequently used. ANG is characterized by a necrosis at the top of the interdental papillae. Later the disease process spreads along the marginal gingiva in the form of punched lesions, as seen in the illustration which is from a 22-year-old woman. The lesions are covered by grayish-yellow pseudomembranes which, when removed, expose a bleeding surface. There is a marked tendency towards bleeding and an extreme tenderness upon the slightest pressure. A characteristic oral fetor is present, and the patients may suffer from regional lymphadenopathy, increased salivation, and elevated temperature. Occasionally, the ANG may be confined to the top of the interdental papillae, the incipient type[415]. There is also a subacute form, sometimes a type of continuation of the untreated incipient form. It should be noted that ANG has a marked tendency to recur unless properly treated, i.e., careful cleaning of the gingiva and teeth.

Acute necrotizing stomatitis

Acute necrotizing gingivitis may spread, either by direct continuation or by contact, to other areas of the oral mucosa. The area usually affected is the buccal mucosa adjacent to the gingiva of the partially erupted mandibular third molar. The location seen opposite, in an 18-year-old woman, is unusual. The palatal gingiva in the maxilla is also severely affected. Acute necrotizing gingivitis or stomatitis is most often diagnosed among young men with poor oral hygiene. It is well known that epidemics of acute necrotizing gingivitis often are observed among troops in wartime[415]. Although the disease has been known for centuries, the exact etiology is still obscure, although it usually is considered as a fusospirochetal lesion with the spirochetes found at the advancing edge of the lesion. However, recent studies have shown that *Bacteroides melanogenicus* subsp *intermedius* plays a more important role than *Fusobacterium*[116]. Although not directly communicable, acute necrotizing gingivitis is transmissible to a susceptible host. Predisposing factors are tobacco smoking, gingivitis, or local trauma. Acute necrotizing gingivitis is extremely rare among children in the western world but quite prevalent among children in developing countries such as India[418], Nigeria, Gambia and Colombia[283].

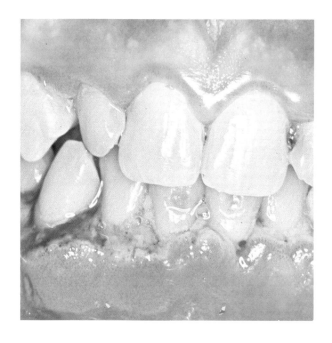

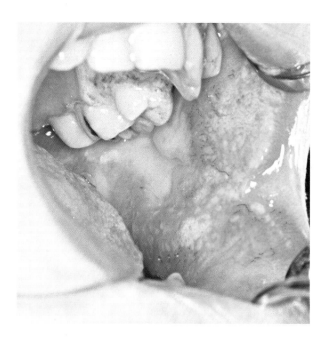

Acute pseudomembranous candidiasis

A variety of oral lesions are caused by the fungus *Candida albicans*, which belongs to the subfamily *Cryptococcoideae*. Previously, the disease was described under names like "moniliasis" and "candidosis", but the general consensus today is that "candidiasis" is a more logical term. Certain factors predispose to the development of candidiasis; any patient receiving antibiotics, corticosteroids, or cytostatic treatment, or suffering from diabetes mellitus, or debilitated from severe systemic disease is more prone to develop candidiasis. The patient seen here was under treatment with corticosteroids and then developed acute pseudomembranous candidiasis (thrush). Acute pseudomembranous candidiasis is characterized by creamy, pearly-white, or bluish-white patches which can be scraped off, leaving an erythematous base. The patches are composed of desquamated epithelium, keratin, fibrin, necrotic tissue, food debris, inflammatory cells, and bacteria heavily infiltrated by hyphae. Thrush favors the buccal mucosa, palate and tongue. In newborns and infants thrush occurs frequently. Prevalences varying from 0.5 to 20 percent have been reported for various nurseries[280]. In a German study it was found that all newborns presenting *Candida* contamination on the seventh day of life were likely to develop a clinically manifest thrush by the end of the second week of life[492].

Acute atrophic candidiasis

The acute candidiasis can be subdivided into an atrophic and a pseudomembranous form, of which the latter is illustrated above. If an acute pseudomembranous candidiasis is not treated it may turn into the acute atrophic variety[324] which, in contrast to the pseudomembranous form, is painful and disturbing to the patient. An acute atrophic candidiasis may be seen as a complication to treatment with broad-spectrum antibiotics and in patients receiving large doses of immunosuppressive and/or cytostatic drugs. The illustration is from the palate of 43-year-old man who suddenly, without any demonstrable cause, developed a fiery reddening of the palate giving rise to a burning and itching sensation. Smears stained with periodic acid-Schiff reagent revealed numerous *Candida*-hyphae. The lesion resolved quickly after local antifungal therapy. Clinically, the acute atrophic candidiasis may resemble the chronic atrophic candidiasis exemplified by a denture stomatitis (p. 62). The chronic type is, however, rarely associated with subjective symptoms. Using cultures of *Candida* for the diagnosis of a possible candidiasis does not seem appropriate as it is known that *Candida* is present as a commensal in the yeast cell form in 50 percent of normal mouths[324].

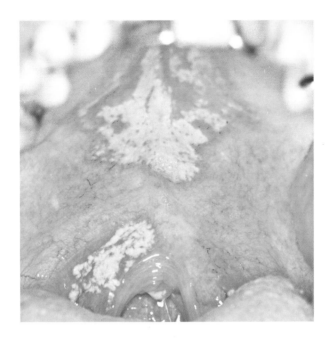

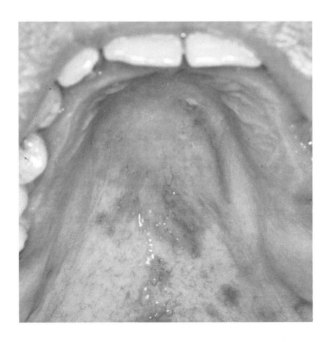

Chronic atrophic candidiasis (angular cheilosis)

The lateral lip fissures, well known among denture wearers, have been called by a variety of names, such as "rhagades", "perlèche", "angular cheilitis", and "angular cheilosis". Previously it was usually accepted that the cause of angular cheilosis was loss of occlusal vertical dimension. It is, however, today generally recognized that the most important factor is infection with *Candida albicans*, coming from an intraoral location, viz., a denture stomatitis[100, 562]. Predisposing factors may be flaccid, sagging cheeks, deepened labial angles constantly moistened by saliva and decreased vertical dimension of the occlusion. Clinically, the condition is characterized by painful fissures radiating from the angles of the mouth. Sometimes there is only one fissure, but most often several small fissures are present. The saliva is seen drooling down in the fissures, which are occasionally covered with yellowish scales, as in the left angle in the 60-year-old woman shown here. Not all investigators agree that *Candida* is the main etiologic factor. *Staphylococcus aureus* has, in one study of angular cheilosis, been isolated almost twice as commonly as *Candida*[347]. When angular cheilosis is present, it should be remembered that the condition may be a manifestation of an iron deficiency anemia.

Chronic hyperplastic candidiasis

Location of a candidal infection at the labial commissure (the retrocommissural area) is more common than previously assumed[279]. Because of its hyperplastic nature the lesion often resembles a leukoplakia, especially the speckled type (p. 196), for which reason the term candidal leukoplakia has been suggested[100]. The commissural candidiasis is usually found in both commissures as in the 47-year-old man pictured opposite, who complained of an itching sensation. He smoked a pipe and 10 cigarettes daily. It is characteristic for the hyperplastic lesion that there are red areas, sometimes the seat of an ulceration. Usually the lesion responds to mycostatic treatment by transforming into a homogenous leukoplakia. Often the commissural candidiasis is part of a multifocal candidiasis affecting the tongue and/or the palate (p. 60). In a British study[279] patients with hyperplastic candidiasis demonstrated a high frequency of both iron and folic acid deficiency, both conditions contributing to the facility with which hyphae of *Candida albicans* penetrate oral epithelium. An early diagnosis and active treatment of a commissural hyperplastic candidiasis is important as there appears to be a definite propensity for malignant change[174].

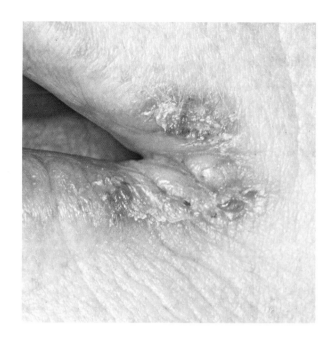

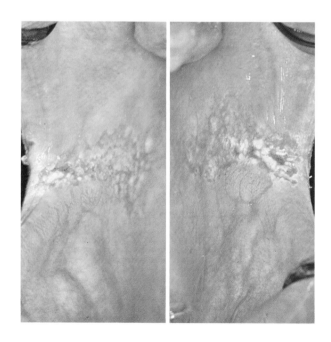

Chronic localized candidiasis on dorsum of tongue

In the first paper on chronic multifocal oral candidiasis[105] attention was called to a lingual location of the candidiasis clinically very similar to the so-called median rhomboid glossitis (p. 218). In a Danish material of 32 patients with chronic multifocal candidiasis 15 were found to have lesions on dorsum of the tongue and 12 of these had a simultaneous palatal lesion[258]. It has been asserted that the palatal and tongue lesions are contact lesions. All these patients were smokers like the 18-year-old man shown opposite. The patient also had a palatal lesion. The smears from both lesions revealed the presence of many fungal hyphae. It is the experience of the author that antifungal therapy can remove the hyphae and change the lesion onto a smooth, whitish, opalescent area. An establishment of normal tongue papillae has not been observed. The relationship between the tongue lesion illustrated and the median rhomboid glossitis has been the object of much discussion in recent years[605]. The area anterior to the terminal sulcus has been suggested to be a locus minoris resistentiae because the vascular supply to the area is very small[302], thus favoring the development of an inflammatory, infectious, or degenerative process[51].

Chronic multifocal oral candidiasis

In 1965 a "candidoses à foyers multiple de la cavité buccale" was described[105] which corresponds to the condition called "chronic hyperplastic candidiasis". The condition, which usually is of long duration, has a predilection for the corners of the mouth, the retrocommissural area, the dorsum of the tongue, and the posterior part of the palate. The lesions consist of white, firm, adherent plaques usually found on an erythematous base, and the clinical appearance may be quite similar to the conditions described in the chronic localized candidiasis or dorsum of tongue (see above) or hyperplastic lesions. Occasionally, the white elements have a nodular appearance, and sometimes they are verrucous. The location on the dorsum of the tongue often corresponds to the area where a median rhomboid glossitis is found. In a Danish material of 32 patients with multifocal candidiasis angular lesions were only seen in denture wearers and only in combination with commissural lesions[258]. The fungal nature of the lesion can be demonstrated by a histologic examination using a periodic acid-Schiff stain, or by response to antimycotic treatment. The illustration opposite demonstrates palatal and lingual lesions in a 65-year-old woman who also had affections of the labial commissures.

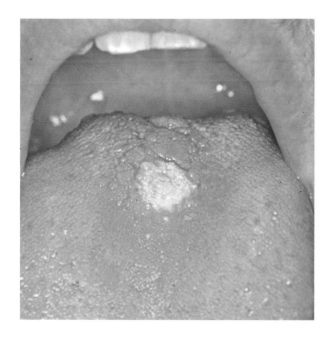

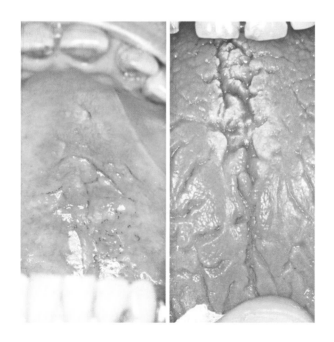

Chronic atrophic candidiasis – denture stomatitis type II

The inflammatory changes seen beneath an upper denture have been called "stomatitis prothetica", "denture sore mouth", or "denture stomatitis" of which the latter term seems to have gained universal acceptance. In selected populations the prevalence of denture stomatitis has been shown[87, 432] to vary from 10 to 65 percent! This very large range in prevalence may be explained by differences in diagnostic criteria or in differences in denture hygiene. Usually the condition is classified into three types: (1) a localized type of inflammation, (2) a generalized simple type of inflammation, and (3) a granular-papillary type[87, 394]. Type I, the local inflammation sometimes called "localized simple inflammation", appears with red spots usually around the small palatal salivary glands (pinpoint hyperemia) and diffuse inflammation of a limited area of the palatal mucosa. This lesion has been reported to be associated with trauma from the dentures. Type II, diffuse reddening, also called "chronic atrophic palatitis", "stomatitis prothetica nudata" or "generalized simple inflammation", appears with a diffuse hyperemic, smooth and atrophic mucosa extending over the entire denture-bearing area[54]. A typical example, in a 43-year-old woman, is seen opposite. Increased growth of yeasts has, among other factors, been associated with this lesion. Therefore, it seems appropriate to use the term chronic atrophic candidiasis.

Chronic atrophic candidiasis – denture stomatitis type III

Type III, the granular or granulated type, also called "inflammatory papillary hyperplasia", "hyperplastic denture stomatitis" or "multiple papillomas of the palate", is characterized by a hyperemic mucosa with a granular or nodular appearance. The granular hyperplasia is usually localized to the central part of the hard palate and may be either nodular or mossy in appearance. The illustration is from a 63-year-old woman with a typical granular denture stomatitis. The symptoms of denture stomatitis are pain, irritation and disturbance of salivation. However, a number of patients with denture stomatitis do not have any symptoms. The etiology of denture stomatitis is multicausal. The significant direct causes of denture stomatitis are infection and mechanical irritation and, less frequently, primary toxic or allergic reactions provoked by constituents of the denture base material. Many studies have related *Candida* to denture stomatitis[87, 93]. Candida hyphae are always present on the denture in cases of denture stomatitis. Poor oral and denture hygiene is a major predisposing condition for Candida-induced stomatitis. Recurrences, despite antifungal therapy, raise the question of whether other factors infrequently studied may be involved in chronic atrophic candidiasis[475].

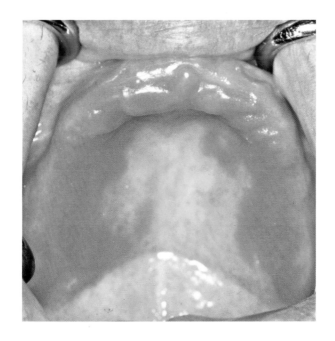

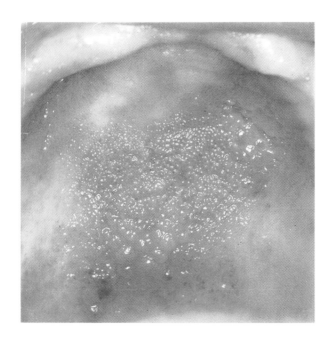

Papillary hyperplasia of palate

The term papillary hyperplasia of palate is usually used for the granular type of denture stomatitis. It should be kept in mind, however, that a papillary hyperplasia may be found also in patients who have a full complement of teeth and who have never worn any type of denture. The condition in dentulous individuals is rare; a survey of 3000 patients presenting for routine prosthetic examination revealed five cases of papillary hyperplasia of palate in patients who had never worn dentures[491]. The illustration opposite, a 38-year-old man who had never worn dentures, is an example of such a case. The lesion characteristically is formed by many ovoid or spherical papilloma-like excrescences 2 to 4 mm in diameter on an erythematous background. Whereas the etiology of papillary hyperplasia in denture-wearers is a *Candida* infection, the cause of the hyperplasia in dentulous persons remains speculative[400]. It seems appropriate, however, to compare the lesion illustrated with the palatal lesions found in the chronic multifocal oral candidiasis (p. 60), where the palatal lesions in some cases have a similarity to the papillary hyperplasia of palate.

Chronic mucocutaneous candidiasis

Chronic mucocutaneous candidiasis (CMC) refers to a heterogeneous group of disorders in which patients suffer prolonged infections of skin, nails, and mucous membranes with *Candida* species, usually *C. albicans*. Associated features may include endocrine disorders and a variety of immunologic deficit[467]. It usually starts early in life, where the oral changes are similar to those seen in acute pseudomembranous candidiasis. Later, however, a deepseated granulomatous process develops. The oral involvement may extend to oropharynx and esophagus, but further visceral extension and sepsis are extremely rare. A subgroup of CMC is the candidal granuloma. It begins in infancy and early childhood often as simple oral thrush and ultimately involves three sites: the oral mucosa, the fingernails and the skin of the face and scalp[22]. The patient shown here, a 13-year-old girl, has an example of a candidal granuloma. The Department has followed the girl since she was 2 years of age. At that age she had lesions of the scalp, the nails and the oral mucosa. In the past 11 years the oral manifestations have undergone changes from rather superficial white patches to deep-seated lesions. The illustration shows how profoundly the tongue is affected.

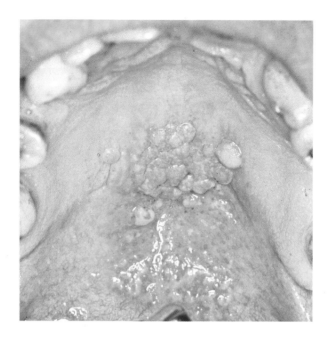

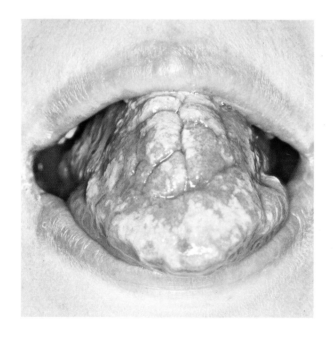

Acquired mucocutaneous candidiasis

Most patients with chronic mucocutaneous candidiasis will have a background of (1) heredity, (2) association with endocrinopathy, (3) late onset in association with malignancy, particularly thymoma, and (4) being of a diffuse variety. However, the patient seen opposite, a 49-year-old man of a very poor general health, appears to have none of the factors mentioned above. He suffers from elephantiasis, cerebral encephalopathy and organic dementia. He developed several large, lobulated, erythematous tumor-like hyperplasias in both commissures, extending onto the skin. Furthermore, he had candidal nail affections and extreme dryness of the oral mucosa which is extremely red due to *Candida* infection. The dryness may be explained by his treatment with sedatives. In patients with acquired mucocutaneous candidiasis like the one described a number of predisposing factors may be involved: iron deficiency and vitamin A deficiency. The skin manifestations may only include angular cheilitis. It is evident from reading the literature that the disease is rare, but also that the group is ill-defined; many cases which have been included in this entity are examples of candidiasis, confined to the oral mucosa, in which a general precipitating factor has been found.

Candida-endocrinopathy syndrome

Chronic mucocutaneous candidiasis may be associated with endocrinopathies involving parathyroids, adrenals, pancreas, thyroid and ovaries. Other components may be observed, such as chronic keratoconjunctivitis, pernicious anemia and enamel hypoplasia[388]. The condition has been called the autoimmune polyendocrinopathy-candidiasis syndrome or the *Candida*-endocrinopathy syndrome[588]. The syndrome is usually evident by the second decade of life. Candidiasis usually precedes the onset of endocrine disorders and starts between months and 14 years of age (average 4 years)[22]. The illustration shows marked palatal affections in a 56-year-old woman with the syndrome. By means of the antigen-antibody crossed electrophoresis, 22 different *Candida albicans* precipitins were demonstrated in her serum[30]. Eight years before admission the patient had a superficial subacute candidiasis of the buccal and palatal mucosa. Gradually the oral condition became worse, with leukoplakic changes developing all over the mouth. The palatal changes are consistent with a speckled leukoplakia with a number of nodular excrescences. Four biopsies from the left buccal mucosa, tongue, uvula, and hard palate revealed epithelial dysplasia.

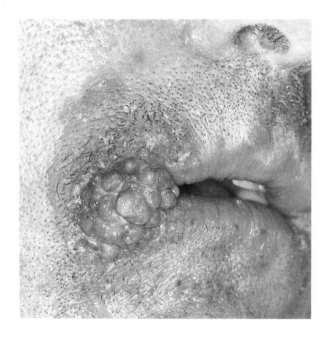

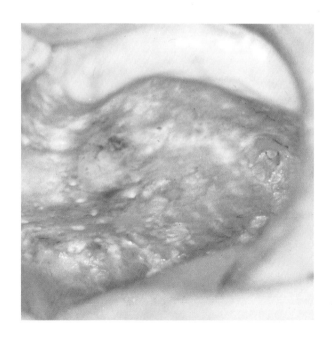

Disseminated histoplasmosis

Histoplasmosis is an infection caused by the *Histoplasma capsulatum*, which grows naturally in soil enriched by the accumulation of either the excreta or feathers of wild or domestic birds or the guano of bats. The infection may occur as an acute pulmonary histoplasmosis, a chronic cavitary pulmonary histoplasmosis, or a disseminated histoplasmosis[184]. The acute type is by far the most frequent. In the disseminated form, multiple organ systems of the body are involved. Usually, mucocutaneous lesions indicate the disseminated type. A review of the literature[53] has revealed 53 reported cases of histoplasmosis with oral manifestations. The oral lesions caused by *Histoplasma capsulatum* may occur as local histoplasmosis or as part of the disseminated form. The oral lesions, which may affect the gingiva, palate, tongue, and oropharynx[442] have an extremely varied clinical picture. The lesions may present as ulcerative, nodular, or vegetative processes, often simulating carcinoma. The ulcerations are deep, with infiltrated edges, and are accompanied by regional adenopathy. The picture illustrates a typical gingival lesion in a 25-year-old man, who developed disseminated histoplasmosis following heavy exposure to dust during the process of renovating an old home. (Courtesy of Dr. B. Radden, Melbourne, Australia).

South American blastomycosis

The South American blastomycosis is caused by *Paracoccidioides brasiliensis*, a fungus which lives in soil and on vegetation. The disease occurs most frequently in Brazil and has been seen in most South American countries; sporadic cases found outside this area have all been in, or have had contacts with products from South America[288]. The infection is most prevalent in young adults, with a strong preference for men. It is acquired from the soil or through lesions caused when twigs are used in dental hygiene or when leaves are chewed. Poor oral hygiene favors the infection. The South American blastomycosis, chronic and usually fatal, may appear in various forms. The primary site most often seen is the oral mucosa, with the gingiva as the favored site. From there it spreads to other areas of the oral mucosa, especially the lips, buccal mucosa, palate, and floor of the mouth[71]. The clinical appearance of the oral lesions is clearly demonstrated in the illustrations, which are from a 48-year-old Brazilian man. The affected areas are erythematous, ulcerated, and granulomatous. A large tongue ulceration caused by *Blastomyces dermatitidis* has been reported from S. Africa[520]. (Courtesy of the late Dr. H. Ebling, Porto Alegre, Brazil).

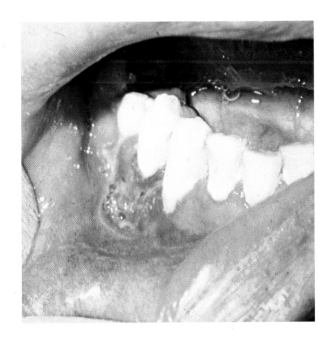

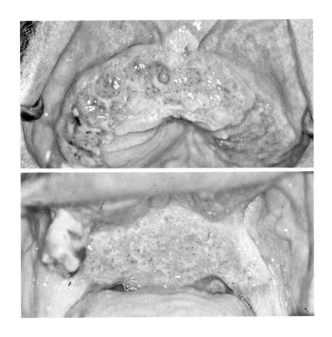

Rhinosporidiosis

Rhinosporidiosis is a fungus infection of the mucosa of the nose, larynx, eyes, ears, and sometimes of the vagina and skin. It is caused by *Rhinosporidium seeberi* and occurs most frequently in India and Sri Lanka, but sporadic cases have been reported from many parts of the world. The disease is probably acquired by bathing or diving into infected water. In India, where rhinosporidiosis reaches epidemic proportions, its rarity in women is attributed to social taboos that prohibit their bathing in open places[73]. Clinically the disease is characterized by the development of friable, highly vascular, sessile or pedunculated polypoid growths, which may be single or multiple. The lesions steadily grow and increase in size. When removed and spread out it has a bundled-up leaf-like appearance. The polyps contain large numbers of globular cysts, sporangia, in various stages of maturity. The sporangium may rupture with release of the spores and cause a corresponding chronic granulomatous reaction with giant cells present[156]. The disease occurs most frequently on the nasal and pharyngeal mucosa, but may also be seen on the palate as in the Indian man, from Kerala in South India, seen here. Also from India is a report of rhinosporidiosis affecting the parotid duct[109]. (Courtesy of the late Dr. J. ZACHARIAH, Trivandrum, India).

Hydatid cyst

The most prevalent of the tapeworms is the *Echinococcus granulosus*, also known as *Taenia echinococcus*. At the larval stage the worm is normally found in sheep, cattle and pigs, but man can become infected with the larval form by contamination with the eggs passed by dogs which have eaten infected feces. When the ova are swallowed by man, the enclosed embryo is liberated in the duodenum. It penetrates the intestinal mucosa, reaches the portal circulation, and is usually held in the liver for 12 hours, where it develops into a hydatid cyst. Alternatively, it may pass the liver filter and reach the lungs and other parts of the body[156]. It develops into a hydatid cyst wherever it eventually comes to rest. A case of hydatid cyst of the tongue is illustrated opposite in a 18-year-old Bantu woman who complained of a painless swelling, present for the previous 3 months, of the right border of the tongue[411]. The unilocular cyst was removed surgically without rupturing, and the hydatid was diagnosed only when the cyst was cut in half and the brood capsules and germinal membrane discovered. A similar case has been reported in a 9-year-old girl from Morocco[549]. (Courtesy of Drs. D. S. C. PROCTER, P. PERL, T. PERL & B. GOLDBERG, Port Elizabeth, South Africa).

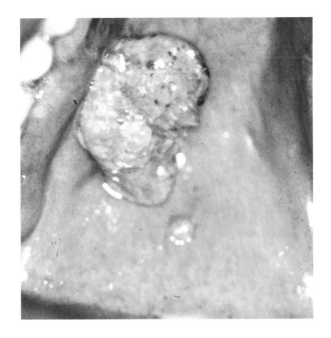

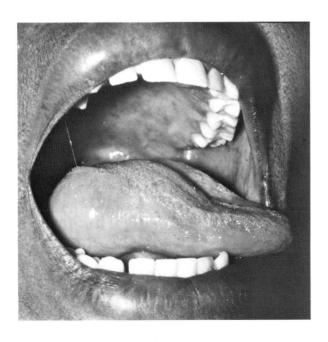

Sarcoidosis

Sarcoidosis, a systemic granulomatous disease of undetermined etiology, has been described under names such as "Besnier-Boeck-Schaumann's disease", "Boeck's sarcoid", and "benign lymphogranulomatosis". Sarcoidosis is one of the diseases which are characterized by an abnormal immune response, mostly expressed by an impaired cell-mediated delayed-type hypersensitivity[574]. The diagnosis is made from a biopsy combined with a positive Kveim test. Sarcoidosis mainly attacks the lungs, lymph nodes, skin, eyes, and bone. Oral manifestations are quite rare. Most often affected are the lips; then, with decreasing frequency, the soft palate, buccal mucosa, gingiva, and tongue. The oral lesions may be solitary or part of generalized sarcoidosis. The patient shown here is a 48-year-old woman who had lung infiltrates and several skin lesions. The lower lip was the site of a nodular swelling of a cartilage-like consistency. The small wound is due to a biopsy. Notice also the typical skin lesions. More often than intraoral lesions, the parotid glands are affected by sarcoidosis.

Behçet's syndrome

The triple symptom complex of Behçet originally comprising oral ulcers, genital ulcers, and iritis now also includes vasculitis, synovitis, gastrointestinal lesions, cutaneous manifestations and meningoencephalitis. The most usual age of onset is between 20 and 30 years and the prevalence is highest in Japan and in countries bordering the Mediterranean. The etiology is unknown. A viral origin has often been postulated but never proven. Immunologic studies have provided indirect evidence that immune complexes are found in the plasma of patients with Behçet's syndrome[594]. Atypical lymphocytes with deep nuclear indentations have been demonstrated by electron microscopy in the prickle cell layer of the oral epithelium of patients with the syndrome[262]. Several studies of histocompatibility antigens have shown an increase in HLA-B5, DR5 and MT2 antigens in patients with the syndrome[401]. The oral lesions are very prominent and they may be the initial manifestation of the disease. The oral ulcers may be located anywhere on the oral mucosa. Morphologically, they resemble aphthae, being well demarcated and varying in size from a few millimeters to a centimeter in diameter. The illustration shows a typical oral lesion in a 23-year-old Turkish man with the syndrome.

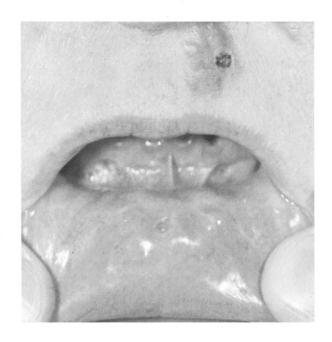

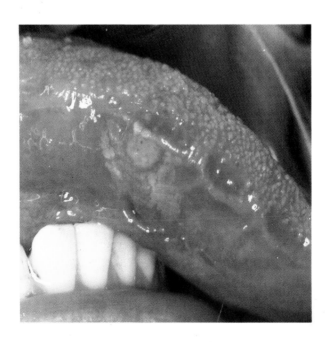

73

Carcinoma of lip (vermilion border)

In the Western world, oral cancer accounts for only 1 to 5 percent of all cancers. In some countries in Southeast Asia, oral cancer represents 15 to 40 percent of all cancers[416]. Also, when specific sites in the oral cavity are considered, marked geographic variations occur. In Western countries, the site most often affected is the vermilion border of the lip, which is only rarely the seat of cancer in dark-skinned people in Asia and Africa[12]. Undoubtedly, melanin acts as a protector by providing a physical barrier blocking the passage of ultraviolet light. The highest annual incidence rates for vermilion border cancer (27, 13 and 12 per 100,000) are found in Newfoundland (Canada), Malta, and Utah (U.S.A.)[585]. Cancer of the lip is a disease which predominantly occurs in men of advanced age. In some countries there is a falling trend in age-adjusted incidence rates for cancer of the vermilion border[381]. By far the most common initial or presenting sign is ulceration. The tumor may present a varied clinical picture from a large exophytic tumor to a deep ulcerative process, as in the 70-year-old man shown opposite. A most important feature is the induration which can be palpated at the periphery of the tumor and which can be seen clearly in the illustration.

Carcinoma of lip (vermilion border) ·

In contrast to the rather dramatic tumor illustrated above, the lesion of the lip shown opposite in a 47-year-old man is rather inconspicuous for a malignant tumor. For 8 months the patient had a small ulcer on the left side of the lower lip causing only minor symptoms. Clinically the lesion presented with crust formation on the vermilion border and a leukoplakia on the labial mucosa. A slight induration could be palpated, and a biopsy revealed a squamous cell carcinoma. It is characteristic that leukoplakias are almost never observed on the vermilion border, which is a dry epithelial surface[416]. A humid environment is necessary for the development of a leukoplakia. Keratoacanthoma should be considered in the differential diagnosis. Most of the larger studies of lip cancer have emphasized the significance of smoking, particularly pipe-smoking. Lip cancer is often preceded by chronic cheilitis of unknown etiology; this is possibly enhanced by an actinic (senile) elastosis supposed to be observed mainly among outdoor workers. The role of actinic radiation as an important etiological basis for lip cancer has, however, been questioned in recent years[332] and a reassessment of these factors has been called for[144, 332].

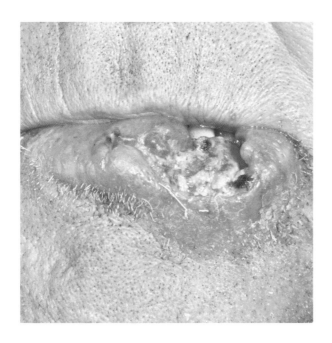

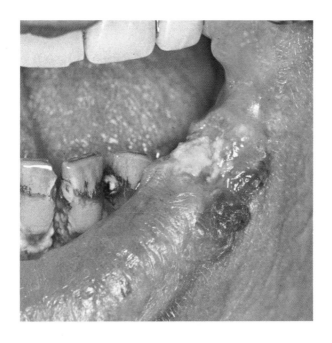

Carcinoma of border of tongue

The incidence of cancer of the tongue shows a considerable variation in a number of countries. The highest incidence rates are found in India (Bombay), Puerto Rico and Brazil (Sao Paulo)[416]. Whereas cancer of the anterior part of the tongue among Europeans is more frequent than cancer of the base of the tongue, the reverse is the case in certain parts of India. Tongue cancer affects men more than women, although this trend is less pronounced in the Scandinavian countries and England than in other countries. However, in the U.S.A., the male:female ratio has decreased rapidly and steadily[268]. The highest incidence of tongue cancer occurs in the sixth to the eighth decades. The symptoms of patients with carcinoma of the tongue depend upon the location of the tumor. When located on the anterior two-thirds, the chief complaint is the presence of mass, which is often painless. When occurring on the posterior one-third the tumor is not always recognized by the patient and the pain experienced is usually attributed to a sore throat. Clinically, tongue cancer may manifest in a variety of ways. Often it is exophytic with indurated margins as in the 67-year-old woman shown here whose carcinoma developed in conjunction with a new denture.

Carcinoma of inferior surface of tongue

In contrast to the large carcinoma illustrated above, the leukoplakic lesion shown opposite is inconspicuous. For 2 months, a 67-year-old man had felt a small swelling on the inferior surface of the tongue. There was also a slight itching sensation during smoking. In the anterior part of the white lesion small nodular excrescences can be recognized. These nodules are important signs of danger and their presence should always lead to a biopsy (see also p. 80, 190 and 196). In the present case the biopsy revealed a squamous cell carcinoma. Leukoplakic patches may be seen in the vicinity of many tongue carcinomas. The majority of growths arise on the lateral borders and undersurfaces of the anterior two-thirds of the tongue, while only one-quarter arises in the posterior third[199]. Using the TNM classification[19] the majority of tongue cancers are 2 cm or more in diameter at the time of diagnosis. Regional lymph node metastasis at the time of admission has been reported at about 50 percent. Patients with tongue cancer are usually heavy smokers and often heavy drinkers. Previously, when tertiary syphilis was rather prevalent, a number of tongue cancers developed in such patients, often preceded by leukoplakic patches.

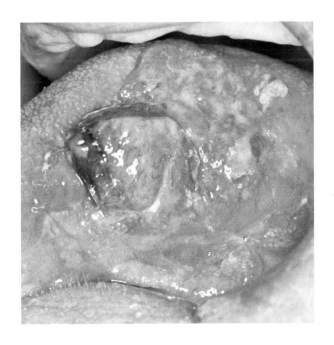

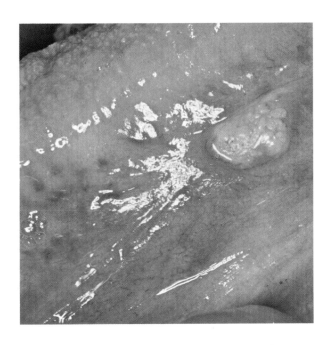

Fibrosarcoma of gingiva

Peripheral fibrosarcoma of the jaws is a rare condition. When it occurs it is most often found inside the bone, called the central or intraosseous type. An example of an unusual peripheral fibrosarcoma originating from the gingiva is illustrated opposite. The patient is a 13-year-old girl who noticed a swelling in the left mandible 4 weeks before admission. When the swelling had been present for 2 weeks she went to her dentist, who removed what he considered to be an innocuous epulis. No histologic examination was done. The lesion recurred, and 2 weeks after the first operation the lesion had grown to the size seen on the picture. The tumor, clinically presenting itself as an "epulis", was soft and sessile. After surgical removal of the tumor, histologic examination showed it to be a low-grade fibrosarcoma with small foci of giant cells of the same type as seen in a giant cell granuloma. A local resection of the underlying bone was done. The rather conservative approach was motivated by reports in the literature that peripheral, circumscribed fibrosarcomas in the jaws of young individuals have a relatively good prognosis. A clinically similar but histologically anaplastic case of a fibrosarcomatous epulis has been reported[193].

Carcinoma of alveolar ridge

The patient shown opposite is an 81-year-old man whose denture had not fitted him well for 2 months. For many years he had been smoking cheroots and cigars. Clinically the lesion presented as a homogeneous leukoplakia in the sulcus but nodular on the alveolar ridge. A radiograph revealed a radiolucent destruction with blurred borders corresponding to the clinical changes. A biopsy showed the lesion to be a squamous cell carcinoma. Despite the fact that the mucosa covering the gingiva and the edentulous alveolar ridge are different in their histologic structure, most investigators do not distinguish between cancer of the gingiva and cancer of the alveolar ridge; they usually use the term "the gums" for both sites. A distinction between the two structures is desirable, as a marked difference in survival rates for the two sites has been demonstrated. In one of the largest samples (606 patients) of gingival (alveolar) carcinomas, from U.S.A.[92], 77 percent were men and 23 percent women. As for other sites, a decrease has been demonstrated in England[152] in the male:female ration for mandibular ridge (gingiva) cancer from the period 1932–9, when it was 5:1 to the period 1960–9, when the ratio was 1:1.

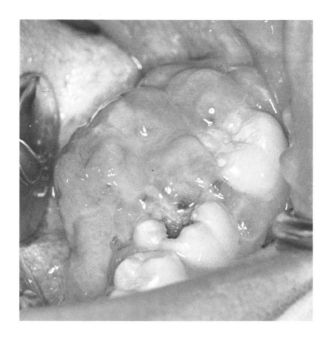

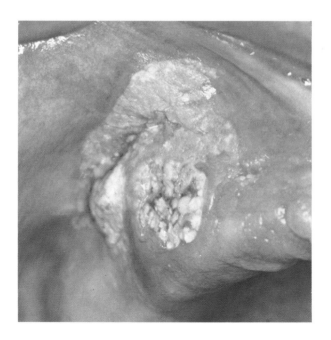

Carcinoma of floor of mouth

Cancer of the floor of mouth accounts for 10 to 15 percent of all oral cancers in the Western world, whereas cancer in this location is rare in Burma, India, and Sri Lanka, where oral cancer incidence is otherwise significantly higher than in the West. Cancer of the floor of mouth is a disease of middle and old age with a peak prevalence in the seventh decade[188]. In some countries there is a marked decrease in the male:female ratio for floor of mouth cancer. Floor of mouth cancer is a clinical entity only in its early stages. Involvement of adjacent structures is common and the disease soon spreads beyond the floor itself. Clinically, the most frequent finding is of an ulcerated lesion with raised and indurated margins located near the lingual frenum. The base of the ulcer presents a reddish-grey, indolent appearing granular surface which ordinarily is free of slough. Sometimes the cancer may present as an inconspicuous white lesion, as in the 17-year-old man shown opposite. In a study of 67 asymptomatic floor of mouth cancers and carcinoma *in situ* it was found that an erythroplakic component occurred in 97 percent[354]. Several studies have demonstrated an association between cirrhosis of the liver and floor of mouth cancer[295]. In a material of 377 patients with floor of mouth cancer 36 percent had cervical metastasis[818].

Carcinoma of labial commissure

Labial commissural cancers are almost always registered as cancers of the buccal mucosa. In doing so, one excludes the possibility of distinguishing between two different points of origin for the cancer, which may have a different etiology. A very frequent site for leukoplakia is the labial commissure and, as some leukoplakias become malignant, quite a number of oral cancers will begin in the labial commissure. This is the case in the patient shown here, a 65-year-old man who had had a bilateral lesion in the labial commissures for several years and who had been smoking excessively for many years. The left lesion had leukoplakic patches and resembled the nodular type of leukoplakia (p. 196). A biopsy revealed a squamous cell carcinoma. As most nodular leukoplakias show the presence of *Candida* hyphae, some investigators have been tempted to consider that some cases of chronic candidiasis may be precancerous lesions. It has been suggested[101] that there may be a strong association between advanced candidal leukoplakia (p. 190) and cancer. Cases of this nature have now been reported. The majority of cancers located on the commissure are well-differentiated squamous cell carcinomas, and they are rather slow-growing tumors.

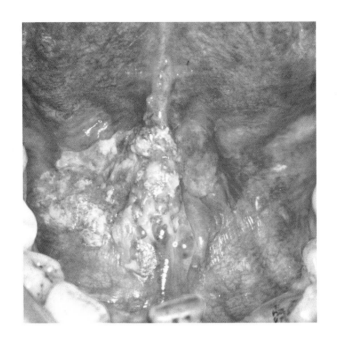

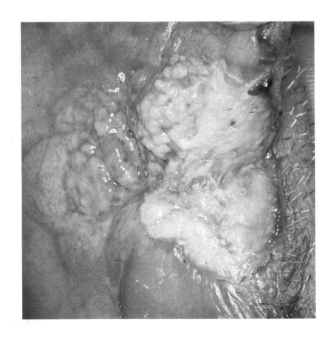

Carcinoma of labial commissure and buccal mucosa

Squamous cell carcinoma of the buccal mucosa in the Western countries is predominantly a disease of the old and very old age groups[575]. The patient opposite is a 55-year-old man from South India. For many years he had chewed a mixture of betel (areca) nut, betel leaves, slaked lime, and tobacco. This quid had been kept in contact with the right and left buccal mucosa for many hours, day and night. The carcinoma affects the labial commissure and the right buccal mucosa, and there is a break-through to the skin. The cancer is red in the center, dominated by red nodules (erythroplakic), and white (leukoplakic) at the periphery. The left commissure is also the seat of a carcinoma. Studies in India have clearly demonstrated that chewing betel nut alone does not cause oral cancer[228]. Only when tobacco is included may malignant disease occur, the location being dependent upon where the quid is habitually held. In most areas of India the quid is normally kept in the lower buccal sulcus. If the quid is retained during sleep the risk of oral cancer developing is 60 times greater than for non-chewers. In areas where chewing tobacco together with betel nut is a widespread habit, annual incidence rates of 21–33 oral cancers per 100,000 have been established[227, 578]. Smoking in various forms in India also increases the risk of oral cancer.

Verrucous carcinoma of buccal mucosa

Cancer of the buccal mucosa (including commissure) accounts for 10 to 15 percent of all oral cancers, and very often is proceded by a leukoplakia, occasionally of papillomatous or speckled nature (p. 196). The patient shown here is a 65-year-old woman with a papillomatous lesion in the right cheek and a leukoplakia outside the lesion. The biopsy revealed a verrucous carcinoma (or Ackerman tumor), a tumor with an expansive more than infiltrative growth and a tumor sometimes difficult to diag-nose[363]. The patient had smoked six cheroots daily for 23 years. A rather frequent occurrence of verrucous carcinomas of the oral mucosa is reported from Papua-New Guinea with the labial commissures and buccal mucosa as the most prevalent locations[123]. It has been suggested that the predilection of the verrucous carcinoma for the labial commissures is related to the repeated application of slaked lime in connection with betel chewing and smoking. The frequency of verrucous carcinoma in materials or oral cancer varies from 2 to 20 percent. In a study of 198 cases of oral verrucous carcinoma[274] it was found that 58 percent were located on the buccal mucosa. Clinically, the tumor is at first relatively soft and circumscribed but it usually becomes firm and more indurated.

82

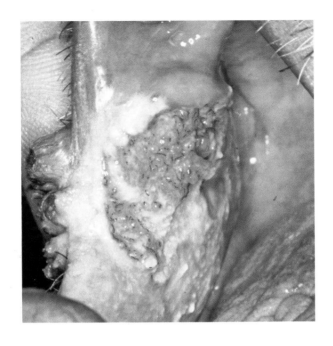

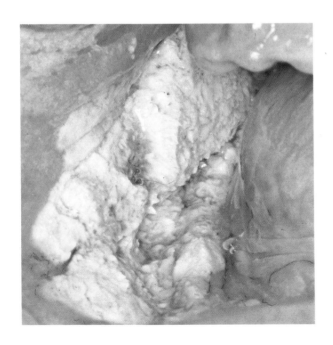

Carcinoma of palate

Whereas palatal squamous cell carcinoma is rather common in countries or areas where the habit of reverse smoking is practiced, palatal cancer is, in most parts of the world, the rarest location of all oral cancers. Adenoid cystic carcinomas derived from the palatal salivary glands are more frequent than squamous cell carcinomas (p. 86). The latter type usually develops laterally in the posterior part of the palate with the majority of cases located on the soft palate[450]. Many lesions appear to develop at or close to the junction of the hard and soft palates[581]. Men are affected three to four times more frequently than are women. Swelling, pain and ulceration are the most frequent symptoms. Patients with poorly-differentiated carcinomas will complain of an ulceration more often than patients with highly differentiated carcinomas[166]. The palatal cancer usually develops as a rather flat swelling, which later ulcerates. This is exemplified in the illustration of a 57-year-old woman, who smoked four cheroots daily. The tumor had developed slowly over a period of 4 years. In a number of cases the cancer is preceded by a leukoplakia but not a smoker's palate (p. 198). Metastasis is found only in one-fourth or one-third of the cases.

Carcinoma of palate in reverse smoker

The patient shown here is an 18-year-old Indian woman who, for the last 10 years, had smoked Indian cherrots with the burning end inside the mouth. The result was an extensive palatal squamous cell carcinoma, ulcerated and with regional lymph node metastasis. The habit of reverse smoking has been reported from South India, the Philippines, Sardinia, Jamaica, Venezuela, Colombia, Panama, and some islands of the South Caribbean. In an area in India where the habit of smoking native cheroots (chuttas) with the lighted end inside the mouth is prevalent, palatal cancer accounts for 45 percent of all oral cancers[452]. In reverse smokers carcinoma of the hard palate usually develops as an ulcer lateral to the midline of the glandular zone of the hard palate. Also in Panama, Sardinia, Colombia, and Venezuela a large number of palatal cancers are found. The precancerous lesions caused by reverse smoking of chuttas have been studied among 10,000 Indian villagers[426]. Fourty-four percent of the population smoked the reverse way, the majority being women, and 18 percent of the habitués showed palatal lesions. In the same population sample an annual oral cancer incidence rate of 22 per 100,000 has been found[227].

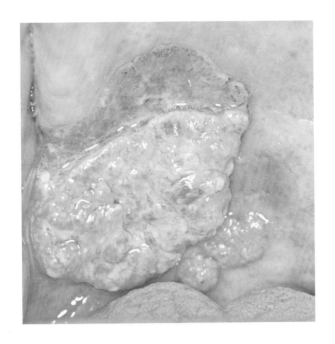

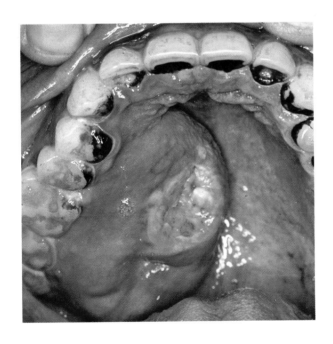

Adenoid cystic carcinoma of palate

Intraoral salivary gland tumors account for 10 to 20 percent of all salivary gland tumors. The most frequent of the malignant intraoral neoplasms of salivary gland origin is the adenoid cystic carcinoma[554] (previously called cylindroma) which makes up about 10 to 30 percent of all palatal salivary gland tumors[165, 461], in contrast to the parotid gland, where the adenoid cystic carcinoma represents only about 2 percent of all the salivary gland tumors. The prognosis is better when the tumor is localized to the palate than to the submandibular or parotid glands[165]. The palatal adenoid cystic carcinoma is a firm and infiltrating tumor, occurring on one side of the midline. Occasionally it is ulcerated, as in the 55-year-old man shown here, and sometimes it is accompanied by pain. The slow growth rate of this neoplasm is apparent from the lengthy periods between the appearance of the first symptom and the diagnosis. Even when radical surgery is performed, the adenoid cystic carcinoma very often recurs and may, in late stages, invade the middle fossa of the skull. Recurrences have been seen in 59 percent of patients with adenoid cystic carcinoma with a tubular pattern, as compared to 89 percent for the cribriform lesions and 100 percent for the solid neoplasms[412].

Metastasis from lung carcinoma

Metastatic lesions to the jaws and oral mucosa constitute 1–8 percent of all the malignant tumors in the oral region[402]. The majority of metastatic lesions to the oral region are intraosseus; only 14 percent are located to the soft tissue of the oral cavity[402]. Among the soft tissue areas the tongue and gingiva are most often the seat of metastatic deposits. The patient shown here is a 65-year-old woman who had experienced pain the left side of the maxilla for 4 months. Two weeks before admission the patient noticed a swellin buccally to the premolars in the same region. Between the two premolars there was a large tumor covering three-fourths of buccal surfaces of the premolars. The tumor was removed and the histologic diagnosis was a low differentiated carcinoma suspicious for metastasis. As the patient had been operated for a lung carcinoma 3 months before admission it was concluded that the "epulis" was a metastasis from the lung tumor. The illustration shows a recurrence observed 2 weeks after the removal of the tumor. In a similar case, recently reported, the gingival swelling was first diagnosed as a pyogenic granuloma, giant cell granuloma or a fibroma[476]. The frequency of oral metastasis from lung malignancies, as percent to the mouth, appears to be increasing.

86

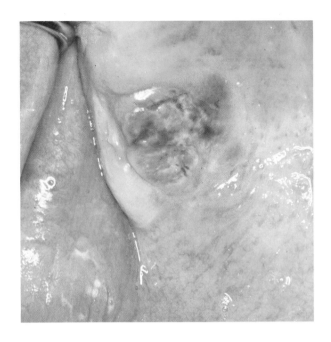

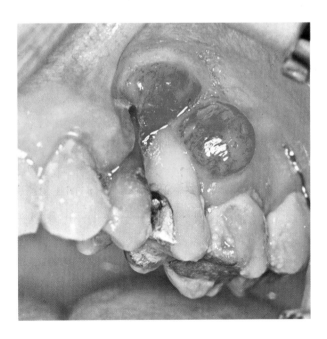

Malignant melanoma of buccal mucosa

Malignant melanoma is a cancerous condition of the melanocyte most often affecting the skin. The frequency of oral location among all melanomas varies from 0.4 to 0.8 percent[335]. The intraoral melanoma, which shows an equal sex distribution, is diagnosed at an average of 58 years[335]. The most common sites for intraoral melanomas are the palate[348], alveolar ridge/gingiva, the buccal mucosa and the lips (vermilion border and labial mucosa). The tumor may present in two different ways. It may either have a short history with rapid enlargement and a very poor prognosis, or may appear as a mass developing in a pigmented area previously present for months or years as a flat plaque and with a much better prognosis, the so-called superficial spreading melanoma (pagetoid melanoma, melanoma *in situ*). The primary intraoral melanoma has a marked tendency for metastases, and the prognosis for this lesion is more serious than for cutaneous melanoma. The patient shown here is a 76-year-old woman who died from distant metastases 4 months after diagnosis and extensive surgery. A possible connection between melanomas and presence of oral pigmentation (melanoplakia) has been reported for Ugandans and Indians[528].

Metastasis from mammary carcinoma

Metastasis from a breast carcinoma is the most frequent type of spread of malignancy to the oral regions. Among 86 such cases, only two were located to the oral soft tissues, the rest having an intraosseous location[402]. The patient shown opposite exemplifies a metastasis to the oral soft tissue simulating an epulis. Six years before admission, the patient, a 62-year-old woman, had an operation for a mammary carcinoma. Five years later there was a recurrence, which was surgically removed. One year later there was another recurrence, a suspicious metastasis in the brain and the lesion illustrated opposite affecting the left tuberosity. A biopsy showed a low differentiated adenocarcinoma thus proving that the lesion was a metastatic deposit as it had the same structure as the original breast tumor. As breast cancer is one of the most common malignant tumors in women it is not surprising that it is the predominating type of tumor metastasizing to the oral regions. When a metastasis from a breast cancer affects the jaws, the mandible is more often affected than the maxilla and the molar area is the preferred site. A similar case has recently been reported[160]. In a Japanese material of 41 metastases to the oral regions 23 cases were located to the gingiva[396].

88

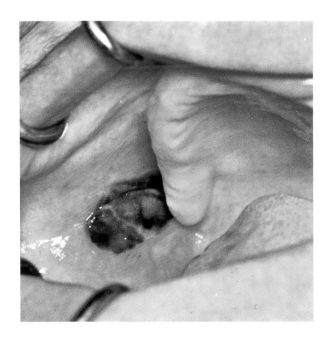

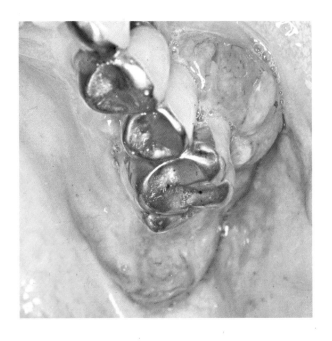

Histiocytic lymphoma

According to the WHO classification[356] the histiocytic lymphoma (HL) (reticulosarcoma) is a malignant tumor composed of large cells of uncertain origin which, when showing evidence of the production of argyrophilic fibrils, or phagocytosis, or both, have been interpreted as neoplastic reticulum cells, histiocytes or other mononuclear phagocytes. HL belongs to the so-called non-Hodgkin's lymphomas. Of a total of 1467 extranodal non-Hodgkin's lymphomas, 417 (28 percent) were in the head and neck region. Of these, tonsils + salivary glands + oral cavity made up 58 percent[200]. In the mouth the palate is the favored location[159]. In the head and neck area the cervical lymph nodes or Waldeyer's ring are usually the sites of origin. A primary extranodal manifestation of HL is rare in the oral mucosa. When it occurs, as in the 71-year-old man seen opposite, the lymphoma presents itself as a well defined soft swelling usually associated with ulceration. In contrast to a squamous cell carcinoma, an HL does not show induration at the periphery of the tumor. The HL with an oral location will most often be characterized by swelling and sometimes ulceration. Most of the cases of intraoral primary HL seen by the author have been located to the palate.

Lymphocytic lymphoma

In the WHO classification "lymphosarcomas" are listed under nodular and diffuse lymphosarcomas (lymphomas). A primary lymphocytic lymphoma (LL) involving the soft tissues of the oral cavity is rare. It may develop wherever lymphoid tissue is present, and throughout the oral soft tissues small aggregations of lymphocytes are found scattered. When it occurs in the oral mucosa the LL is most often located to the palate[70, 558], although several cases have been reported originating in the gingiva. In some patients a pericoronitis has been the first manifestation of an LL[64]. In a material of eight palatal LL, no destruction of the underlying bone could be detected[70]. The oral LL may be a solitary lesion or, more often, become a widespread disease. The patient shown here is a 76-year-old man who had a bilateral palatal swelling of 1 year's duration. A biopsy of a swollen lymph node at the lower pole of the left parotid gland revealed a diffuse LL. A clinicopathologic entity has been reported under the name of lymphoproliferative disease of the hard palate, which is believed to be malignant or potentially malignant[558]. Another, benign, lesion of the palate: follicular lymphoid hyperplasia is an important differential diagnosis[607].

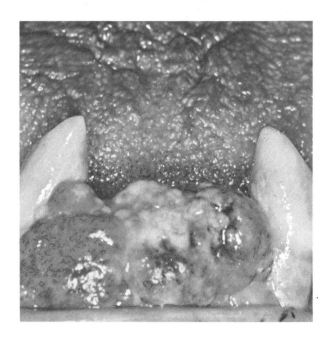

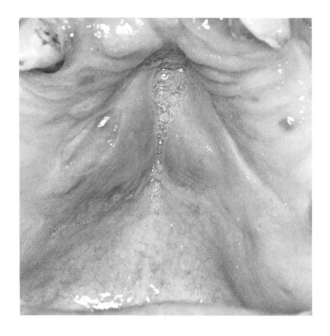

Burkitt's lymphoma

In the WHO classification[356] Burkitt's lymphoma is defined as a malignant neoplasm (a diffuse lymphosarcoma) composed of lymphoid cells believed to be of B-cell type with intensive cytoplasmic basophilia and many sudanophilic cytoplasmic inclusions. Since Burkitt, in 1958, described the entity later to carry his name, multiple malignant neoplasms frequently affecting the jaws[6] but also involving the orbit, ovaries, kidneys, adrenals and other organs to a variable extent, numerous papers have been concerned with the entity among African children. The disease has been the subject of extensive research as it appears to be a tumor of viral origin. The Epstein-Barr (EB) virus has been cultured from jaw tumor cells in patients with Burkitt's tumor[140]. Intense malaria acting over a long period is known to be immunodepressive. It is now accepted that the EB virus in the presence of immunodepression is oncogenic[90]. Burkitt's lymphoma occurs sporadically outside tropical countries. The illustration shows a marked tumor in an 11-year-old Danish girl, who had similar lesions in two other areas of the mouth. A biopsy revealed a Burkitt's lymphoma in this girl who had never been outside Denmark[485].

Hodgkin's disease

Hodgkin's disease (malignant lymphogranulomatosis) is a fatal, systemic disease characterized by a painless enlargement of the lymph nodes and reticuloendothelial system accompanied by fever, anemia, pruritus, and weight loss. The neoplastic element is represented by the typical Sternberg-Reed cells and mononuclear cells with corresponding nuclear features in which a variety of inflammatory cells are intimately associated with the malignant cellular proliferation[356]. The peak incidence of Hodgkin's disease occurs in the second and third decade, and men are affected more often than women. Swollen cervical lymph nodes may be the first manifestation of the disease, and the tonsils also are often enlarged in the initial stages, usually unilaterally. Only a few reports have dealt with oral manifestations, which apparently have a varied picture. Soft tissue swellings of the oral mucosa, sometimes associated with ulcerations and denudation of underlying bone, may occur[49]. The 61-year-old man shown here noticed, 1 month before hospitalization, that there was a loss of retention of his upper denture because of a soft tissue swelling in the palate. A biopsy revealed Hodgkin's disease. No bony involvement could be demonstrated, and the patient was referred for radiation therapy.

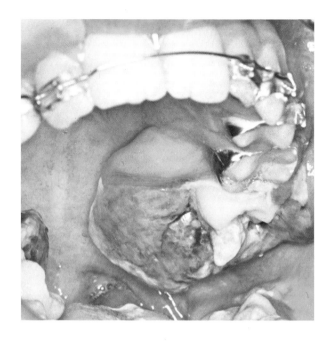

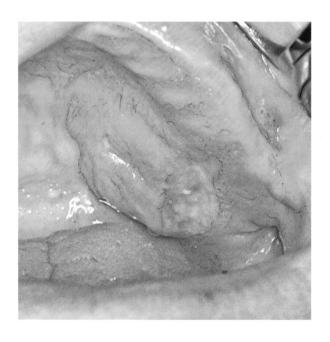

Mycosis fungoides

Mycosis fungoides is a malignant lymphoid neoplasm that always originates in the upper dermis and is characterized by a pleomorphic cellular infiltrate, probably of the T-cell type[356]. It is a systemic condition which almost always ends fatally. Clinically there are four stages of the skin lesions: (1) the premycotic stage; (2) the plaque stage; (3) the tumor stage and (4) spreading to lymph nodes and internal organs. Oral manifestations are rare and most often found in the terminal stage of the disease. The most frequent site for oral manifestations is the tongue. Other sites like palate, buccal mucosa and gingiva may also be affected[606]. In the initial stages the oral mucous membrane may be the seat of erythema which sometimes is extensive and ulcerated[94, 319]. Plaque formation may also occur. Later, smaller and larger infiltrates and tumors appear. The fungus-like lesions may also be grayish-yellow, and sometimes occupy most of the tongue surface. The illustration is of an 75-year-old man who had suffered from enlargement and ulcerations of the tongue for the previous 5 months. During the same period the patient had red-violet spots on the skin. The tongue lesions caused great pain due to extensive ulcerations. A biopsy of the tongue gave the diagnosis of mycosis fungoides.

Chronic leukemia

Leukemia is a malignant disease characterized by a progressive overproduction of any of the white blood cells. In most cases of leukemia, the white blood cells appear in the circulating blood in immature forms. Leukemia is classified into acute and chronic forms, the differentiation between them being related to the degree of anaplasia of the malignant cells, the rapidity of onset, the severity of symptoms and the age of the patient. The acute leukemia of childhood is usually lymphoblastic (ALL). The other acute leukemias can be subdivided into myeloblastic, monoblastic, myelomonocytic, and promyelocytic types. It is, however, convenient to group them together as acute myelogenous leukemia (AML)[437]. Chronic leukemia has an insidious development, shows few clinical signs and symptoms until the disease is quite advanced, and is usually found in adults. Oral manifestations in leukemia are much more common in the acute than in the chronic forms. Mucosal pallor, prolonged bleeding after extraction, and mucosal petechiae may be observed in patients with chronic leukemia. Also superficial ulcerations of the oral mucosa can be seen. The two palatal ulcerations in the illustration opposite were found in a 24-year-old man who had had a chronic myeloid leukemia for 4 years.

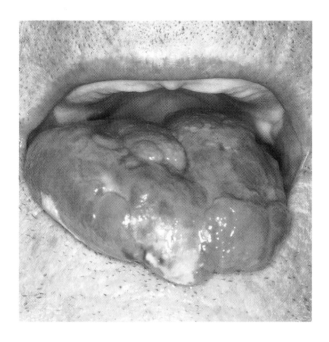

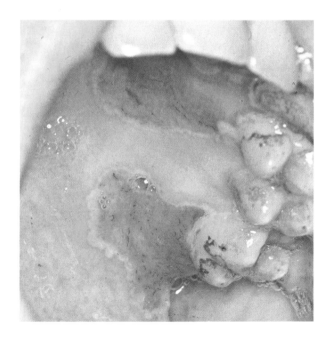

Acute leukemia

Sometimes the tumor cells in the acute forms of leukemia are so immature that they defy classification. The term "stem cell leukemia" is then used. Oral manifestations are more frequent in acute leukemia than in the chronic form. In patients with acute leukemia, oral signs lead to the diagnosis equally as frequently as extraoral signs[344]. It should be emphasized, however, that oral signs may be lacking entirely. Most frequent is lymphadenopathy of the cervical and submandibular regions. In a group of 34 children, 68 percent had palpable cervical lymph nodes at the initial examination[591]. Other manifestations of dental interest are ulcerations, gingival enlargement, spontaneous gingival bleeding, and mucosal petechiae and ecchymoses. In contrast to the rather superficial and limited ulcerations in patients with chronic leukemia, the ulcerations seen in acute leukemia may be extensive and deep, as in the illustration from a 70-year-old man, who had an acute myeloid leukemia. Ulcerations or areas of necrosis of the oral mucosa in patients with leukemia may be explained as the result of: (1) defective defense mechanisms, so that minor traumas may have a serious effect; (2) a thrombosis of the small blood vessels due to the large atypical cells, with subsequent infarction.

Acute leukemia

In a sample of 1076 adult patients with acute leukemia the frequency of leukemic gingival enlargement was 3.6 percent. In another American study of 52 patients with acute leukemia, 38 percent had oral symptoms at the time of diagnosis of the leukemia, but 69 percent had oral signs of leukemia on examination[344]. In the same material 33 percent of the patients had gingival enlargement presumably due to leukemia. This high frequency of gingival enlargement is in contrast to findings in leukemic children where only 10 and 17 percent had gingival enlargement[128, 374]. The enlargement of the gingiva in patients with acute leukemia may be so marked that the teeth may be almost completely covered. The leukemic gingival enlargement is characterized by a shiny, edematous, and boggy appearance. The enlargement seen in leukemic patients may be due to presence of leukemic infiltrates consisting of extravasated and proliferating monocytoid or myeloid cells[147]. The illustration shows a marked enlargement of three interdental papillae associated with ecchymoses in a 39-year-old woman with acute myeloid leukemia. One month before admission she had a swelling of the gingiva, followed later by extensive bleeding. Leukemic infiltrates may also be found in other parts of the oral mucosa.

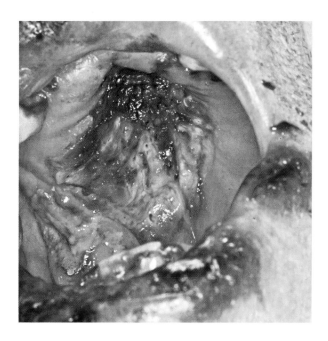

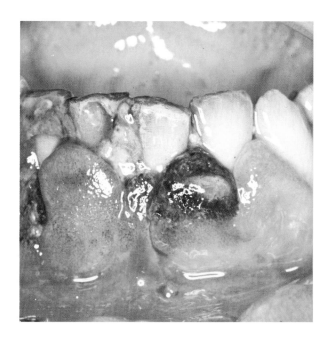

Acute leukemia

The gingival enlargement found in leukemia may sometimes assume monstrous proportions, as in the 44-year-old woman pictured opposite. For 2 months she suffered from a scaling eczema and considerable fatigue. Then her gingiva became swollen and began to bleed spontaneously. At admission she had enlarged lymph nodes and the gingiva was the seat of a most unusual enlargement, as can be seen from the illustration. In several places small petechiae and ecchymoses could be seen. Examination of the blood revealed leukocytes: 65,800/mm^3; differential count: 82 percent immature white cells, 8 percent neutrophils, 10 percent lymphocytes; hemoglobin: 5.6 mg/100 ml; thrombocytes: 40,000, indicating the presence of a stem cell leukemia and secondary anemia and thrombocytopenia. After treatment with a cytostatic drug the enlargement of the gingiva regressed completely[61]. Since cytostatic drugs were introduced in the treatment of leukemia it has become difficult, in some cases, to distinguish between oral changes, especially ulcerations, caused by the leukemia and those produced by the drugs[43]. Also oral hemorrhages may be associated with chemotherapy. In one sample[146] 15 percent manifested gross bleeding from the mouth during the course of treatment.

Monocytic leukemia

Monocytic leukemia is one of the more rare forms of leukemia, but it is often associated with oral manifestations. The illustration opposite shows a fiery red enlargement of the gingiva in a 41-year-old woman in whom a tentative diagnosis of leukemia was made on the basis of the gingival changes seen in the picture. Later, laboratory findings revealed an acute monocytic leukemia. On the top of the interdental papilla between the two mandibular central incisors there is a small ecchymosis. The presence of petechiae or ecchymoses in conjunction with a gingival enlargement is almost pathognomonic for leukemia. The petechiae and ecchymoses are an expression of the secondary thrombocytopenia which so often is found in leukemic patients. In acute promyelocytic leukemia – a variant of AML with extensive hemorrhagic diathesis, fibrinogenopenia, unresponsiveness to therapy, and a rapid, fatal outcome – there is a higher incidence and severity of oral bleeding than in other types of acute leukemia[550]. An almost universal oral feature in patients with acute leukemia is a marked pallor of the oral mucosa due to a secondary anemia usually found in these patients. More unusual oral manifestations in leukemia are numbness or dryness of the oral mucosa.

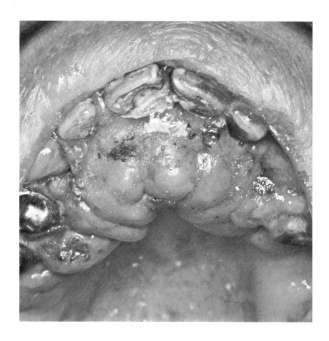

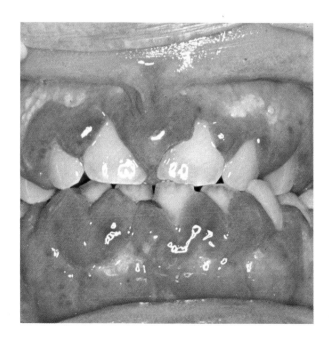

Acute erythremic myelosis

This disorder, also known as Di Guiglielmo's syndrome, or erythroleuke-mia, is characterized by a generalized proliferation of the erythropoietic cells of the bone marrow, similar to the leukocytic proliferation in leuke-mia. The blood contains erythroblasts in all stages of maturation, but the most immature forms are found in disproportionately large numbers[548]. Clinically, there is a severe, rapidly developing anemia, irregular, usually remittent fever, marked splenomegaly, enlargement of the liver, and an acute, ultimately fatal course associated with hemorrhagic manifestations. The clinical course is very similar to that of an acute myeloid leukemia. However, in contrast to leukemia the lymph nodes are rarely enlarged. Also oral involvement appears to be more unusual than in leukemia. The picture illustrates a gingival enlargement and some necrotic interdental papillae in a 28-year-old woman with an acute erythremic myelosis. The clinical appearance is similar to the gingival changes observed in leukemia. After initial symptoms of a sinusitis and anemia, the diagnosis was established through the demonstration of a large number of immature erythrocytes. On the attached gingiva there are small areas of bleeding caused by a secondary thrombocytopenia.

Papilloma of palate

Papillomas originating from surface epithelium are not too common in the oral cavity. They occur at any age, with women slightly more affected than men. They may be found in all intraoral locations, but most commonly on the tongue. With decreasing frequency the papilloma is then found on the palate, buccal mucosa, gingiva and lip[222]. Usually, the tumor is pedunculated, although sessible types also are observed, and a white, sometimes grayish, color is characteristic. The papilloma is made up of many small, finger-like projections, giving the tumor a cauliflower-like appearance. It usually is well circumscribed, but rarely attains a large size. Papillomas are slow-growing and almost always remain benign. Clinically, the papilloma is indistinguishable from the virus-induced verruca vulgaris (viral wart, p. 40). Histologically, the papilloma is covered by a stratified squamous epithelium exhibiting a marked hyperorthokeratosis. Papillomas may be caused by local irritation. In the illustrated case of a 67-year-old man, however, there was no demonstrable cause for the development of the papilloma. A special entity is the papillary hyperplasia of palate (p. 64). Multiple oral papillomas may demonstrate a positive reaction for papilloma virus genus-specific antigens[281].

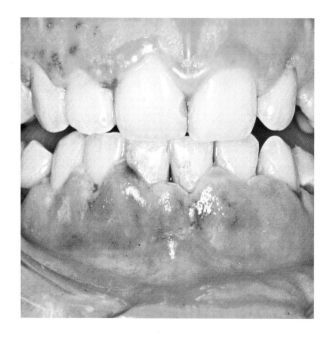

BENIGN NEOPLASMS

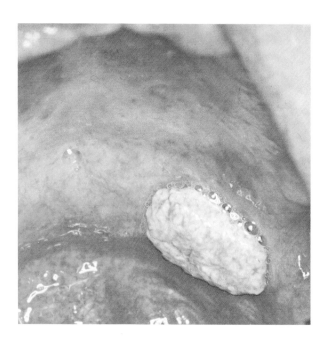

Verrucous hyperplasia of oral mucosa

The entity verrucous carcinoma, or Ackerman's tumor, is well documented. There is, however, another lesion which resembles verrucous carcinoma both clinically and histologically and is frequently mistaken for it and sometimes described as florid oral papillomatosis. The name verrucous hyperplasia is suggested for the lesion, which occurs in elderly people with most cases found in the sixth, seventh and eighth decades with almost the same distribution[512]. Most of our cases involved the gingiva/alveolar mucosa and cheek, followed by tongue, floor of mouth, labial mucosa and palate. In a material of 68 patients, two clinical patterns have emerged[512]. The first, the "sharp" variety, comprises long, narrow, heavily keratinized verrucous processes. The second variety, the "blunt" variety, consists of verrucous processes which are broader and flatter and not heavily keratinized. It is this variety which is illustrated opposite in an 85-year-old woman, who also suffered from benign mucous membrane pemphigoid. The majority of our cases were smokers. In 66 percent of the 68 cases there was associated dysplasia. A recent study[526] has concluded that verrucous hyperplasia probably represents a morphologic variant of verrucous carcinoma.

Monomorphic adenoma – adenolymphoma of buccal mucosa

Monomorphic adenomas are benign growths in which the epithelium forms a very regular, usually glandular pattern, and in which there is no evidence of the mesenchyme-like tissue that is so characteristic a component of pleomorphic adenoma[553]. The term monomorphic adenoma should only be used as a group designation[204]. Adenolymphoma (Warthin's tumor) is characterized histologically by two components: epithelium and lymphoid tissue. The epithelial lining may or may not show a papillary arrangement. The cytoplasm of the epithelial cells is highly eosinophilic (oncocytic cells). The lymphoid component is seen in the supporting stroma and lymphoid follicles are usually present. Normally the adenolymphoma is found in the parotid gland but a few cases have been reported in the intraoral salivary glands[457]. Of the 11 cases reported so far, nine have been in men and two in women, following the pattern known from the parotid gland. The most frequent intraoral locations are the buccal mucosa, the palate, and the labial mucosa[176]. A 67-year-old man was referred for two small bluish nodules in the right buccal mucusa with a diameter of 2 and 4 mm. The lesions showed histologically typical features of an adenolymphoma.

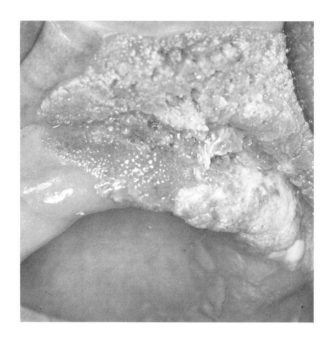

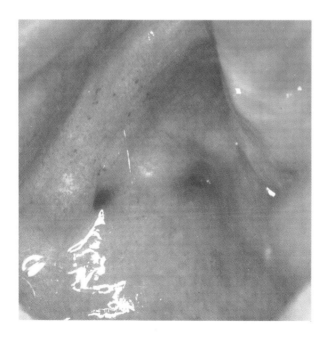

Monomorphic adenoma – sialoadenoma papilliferum of retromolar area

In 1969 a new entity of salivary gland tumors was described[2] under the name of sialoadenoma papilliferum. Since then the tumor has also been called papilliferous cystadenoma. It is a rare, benign and exophytic tumor of the salivary glands. In 1981 nine cases were published, the majority developing in men older than 40 years[390]. The palate has been the commonest site of occurrence. The sialoadenoma papilliferum is an asymptomatic and slow-growing tumor which shows papillary and exophytic proliferation of ductal epithelium with a concomitant overgrowth of surface epithelium. There has been some discussion whether the lesion may represent a focal hyperplasia of duct epithelium rather than true neoplasm[390]. Histologically, the tumor is characterized by a papillary proliferation covered either totally or partly by squamous epithelium. The patient shown here is a 66-year-old man who had an asymptomatic swelling distal and lingual to the right third molar region. Clinically, there was a suspicion of a pleomorphic adenoma. However, the histologic examination of the excised tumor revealed a sialoadenoma papilliferum.

Monomorphic adenoma – basal cell adenoma of upper lip

The basal cell adenoma was first described[301] in 1967 as an entity among the benign salivary gland tumors. However, since that time a disturbing terminologic confusion has been apparent in the literature[204], the reason being that the basal cell adenoma, or basaloid adenoma as it is also called[50], may present with different patterns. Usually four types are recognized (1) solid, (2) trabecular, (3) tubular, and (4) membranous[204]. The basal cell adenoma makes up 15 percent of all intraoral salivary gland tumors in an English material[435]. In a French material[74], the monomorphic adenomas (most of which are basal cell adenomas) make up 12 percent. The basal cell adenoma has a predilection for the upper labial mucosa[328, 502] in distinct contrast to the pleomorphic adenoma most commonly seen in the palate. The basal cell adenoma is an encapsulated, slow-growing, purely epithelial neoplasm composed of apparent basal cells arranged in solid nests, trabecular cords, or tubular patterns. The patient shown opposite was a 66-year-old woman who had a well-demarcated tumor 15 mm in diameter of the upper lip. The lesion was surgically removed and the histologic examination revealed a basal cell adenoma of the trabecular type.

104

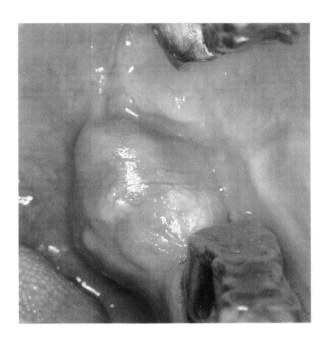

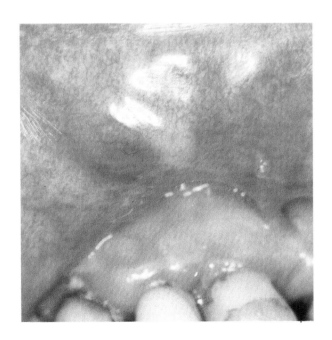

Pleomorphic adenoma of palate

The most frequent of the salivary gland tumors is the pleomorphic adenoma, in both the major and the minor intraoral salivary glands. The tumor is also known under the term "mixed tumor", but it is now generally recognized that only the epithelial element is neoplastic, the others representing metaplastic stroma[554]. In a sample of 1,639 pleomorphic adenomas from salivary glands[164] 6 percent were found in the palate. It is generally agreed upon that the palatal glands are more frequently involved (75 percent)[270], than any of the other groups of minor salivary glands. Among the minor intraoral salivary glands, the pleomorphic adenoma has a palatal location in 60–70 percent[110, 270]. The incidence is highest in the third decade. The most common and consistent symptom is a painless swelling. Not uncommonly, inability to wear dentures is the symptom which brings the patient to the dentist. The tumor usually is found in the posterior part of the palate, as in the 47-year-old woman shown here. The pleomorphic adenoma, which has a slow intermittent growth, is encapsulated, well-demarcated, soft to firm in consistency, and covered by normal oral mucosa, although ulcerations may be seen. The underlying bone may be involved because of pressure from the tumor.

Mucoepidermoid tumor of retromolar area

According to the WHO classification of salivary gland tumors, a mucoepidermoid tumor is characterized by the presence of squamous cells, mucous-secreting cells, and cells of intermediate type[554]. Although the tumor must be regarded as potentially malignant, only a small minority do eventually metastasize. In a series of 331 minor salivary gland tumors (malignant in 55 percent), the mucoepidermoid tumors were the most frequent (22 percent) of the malignant tumors after the adenoid cystic carcinoma[113]. The mucoepidermoid tumor was much more common in women than in men and was found at a greater age than pleomorphic adenoma. The clinical appearance of the lesions varies from bluish to yellow fluctuant masses, to smooth nodules of normal color. An example of an intraoral mucoepidermoid tumor is illustrated opposite. It is in an 82-year-old woman who, 8 months before admission, went to her dentist because her lower denture did not fit due to a swelling. At admission a well-demarcated, soft swelling was found in the right retromolar area. In the center of the tumor there was a faint bluish tinge. A radiographic examination failed to show osseous involvement. A biopsy revealed a highly differentiated mucoepidermoid tumor.

106

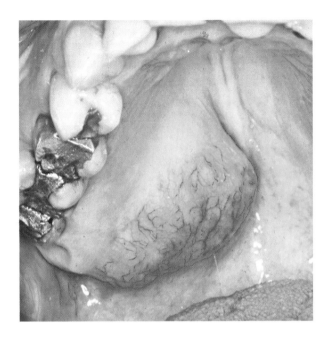

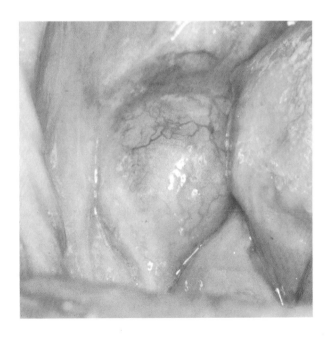

Fibroma of buccal mucosa

The most common tumor of the oral mucosa is the fibroma, which is a benign connective tissue tumor. There is, however, considerable disagreement as to the classification of this lesion. Most authors[341] agree that the so-called oral fibromas are in fact hyperplasias or reactive proliferations of fibrous tissue. In an analysis[41] of 650 localized fibrous lesions from various parts of the mouth, only two lesions were found that could be considered, at least on histologic grounds, to be true fibromas. Most of the so-called fibromas are located on the buccal mucosa and tongue and are definitely caused by irritation. The tumor illustrated opposite, in the buccal mucosa of a 34-year-old woman, could easily be explained as a result of traumatic influence. Fibromas may be found in any area of the oral mucosa. Usually, they are firm, well-demarcated, sessile or pedunculated, and covered by a normal-appearing mucosa. Occasionally, the lesions are covered by a whitish mucosa, indicating a hyperkeratosis. The fibroma rarely causes disturbing symptoms unless it becomes traumatized and thereby ulcerated. Fibromas may also arise from the gingiva in the form of an epulis. These lesions have a tendency for recurrence.

Lipoma of floor of mouth

As lipomas are benign lesions, few are reported but many are seen. A total of 145 cases of oral lipomas appeared in the literature[239] from 1945 to 1967. A lipoma is a benign neoplasm of adipose tissue; it is slow-growing and painless. In the oral mucosa a lipoma is seen most often in the fourth or fifth decade. The most frequent site is the buccal mucosa; thereafter followed by the tongue, the floor of the mouth, buccal sulcus and vestibule, palate, lips, and gingiva. Most reports claim either an overall equal sex distribution or a slight predominance in men[446]. Oral lipomas appear as submucosal, well-defined, round or oval tumors which have a sessile or pedunculated attachment. The surface of an oral lipoma is smooth; the consistency is soft, sometimes with a pseudofluctuation. Therefore, with a sublingual location a careful distinction between a lipoma and a mucocele (p. 174) should be made. As fat is yellow and the overlying epithelium usually is atrophic, the oral lipoma has a characteristic yellowish appearance. The case illustrated is a typical lipoma in the floor of the mouth of a 76-year-old woman. Among the variants of lipomas, several cases of myxoid lipoma have been reported from the oral cavity[112].

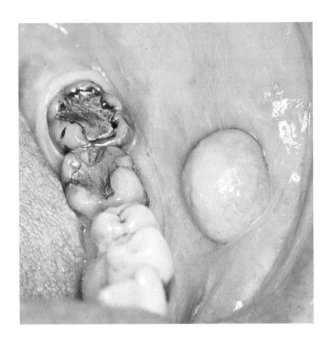

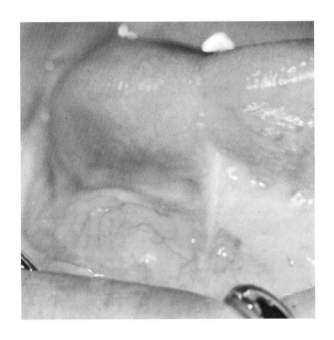

Neurilemoma of tongue

Neurilemoma, also called schwannoma or neurinoma, is a quite rare, benign tumor of nerve sheath origin, apparently derived from the Schwann cells. The tumor, which may arise from any myelinated nerve, usually is solitary, but multiple cases have been reported[126]. In some cases a mechanical trauma has preceded the development of the tumor. In the period 1945 to 1964, 106 cases were reported. There seems to be a preference for the second and third decade[240]. The tongue is the most frequent site for an intraoral neurilemoma; much less commonly affected are the palate, floor of the mouth, buccal mucosa, gingiva, lips, and vestibular mucosa. Usually, the neurilemoma occurs in the mobile portion of the tongue, as in the 23-year-old woman shown opposite. The tumor may present itself as a submucosal nodule, or as a dome-like projection from a mucosal surface. It is generally well-defined and firm in consistency. In the majority of cases the neurilemoma does not cause any disturbing symptoms and the tumor is detected only because of the swelling. The tumor may clinically resemble a salivary gland tumor or a mucocele.

Vascular leiomyoma of gingiva

Leiomyoma is a tumor rarely seen in the oral mucosa because of the paucity of smooth muscles in the oral cavity. Among 7748 benign smooth-muscle tumors of the whole body, only five were from the mouth[180]. This low prevalence is in contrast to the frequent occurrence of leiomyomas in the uterus. When found in the oral mucosa, the leiomyoma most commonly affects the tongue. The next most frequent sites are the buccal mucosa, hard palate and lower lip. The age range shows an even distribution except for a peak between 41 years and 60 years of age[245]. There is no sex predilection. The tumor does not cause pain, and is noticed only because of its mass. The leiomyoma is a slow-growing, well-defined, movable, and firm tumor. Sometimes it is pedunculated. The color of the leiomyoma varies from bluish to reddish, depending on the amount of vessels present. The chief source of smooth muscle is the tunica media of the walls of blood vessels. Therefore, the vascular leiomyoma or angiomyoma is the predominant histologic type[391]. The picture opposite is from a 20-year-old woman who had what was called an epulis. The histologic examination showed it to be a vascular leiomyoma. It is rather unusual in that the tumor is ulcerated.

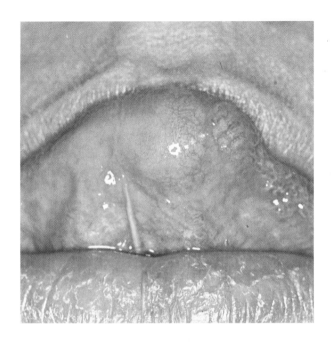

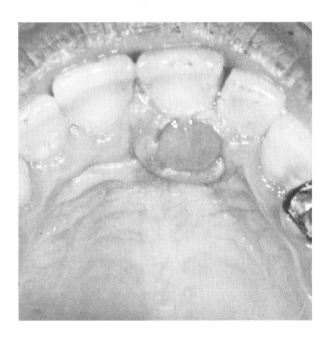

Granular cell myoblastoma of tongue

The granular cell myoblastoma, also known as Abrikossoff's tumor or myoblastic myoma or granular cell tumor, is a benign tumor which occurs in a wide variety of visceral, mucosal, and cutaneous sites, with about one-third located on the tongue. The granular cell myoblastoma occurs in patients of all ages, and there is in some materials a predominance of women. In our own[601] sample of 14 oral granular cell myoblastomas the female:male ratio was 9:4. When located on the tongue the lateral border is the favored site. The tumor also may be seen in other parts of the oral mucosa. Typically, the granular cell myoblastoma is symptomless. Usually the tumor is a small, circumscribed, firm, solitary nodule. A multiple occurrence is estimated to arise in 7–16 percent of all granular cell myoblastomas. A number of granular cell myoblastomas have a whitish surface, which in some cases is due to a pseudoepitheliomatous hyperplasia of the epithelium overlying the tumor. The whitish almost leukoplakic appearance is present in the granular cell myoblastoma illustrated opposite in a 48-year-old man. A preoperative diagnosis of a granular cell myoblastoma is difficult to make, especially for the inexperienced.

Granular cell myoblastoma of tongue

The illustration opposite shows a granular cell myoblastoma from a 54-year-old man. The lesion is larger than the one illustrated above and it does not have the intense white appearance that the other has. It has been suggested that these tumors are derived from Schwann cells, perineural fibroblasts, primitive mesenchymal cells[358], or even histiocytes. Recently, the presence of S-100 protein in granular cell tumors has supported the idea that these tumors arise from Schwann cells[533]. In the Danish material mentioned above[602] all 14 lesions were treated by local excision. In spite of a possible inadequate removal of 10 of the lesions where granular cells extended to the margin of excision, no recurrence was seen in a follow-up period averaging 7 years. Malignant granular cell tumors are rare, making up only 1–3 percent of all reported granular cell tumors. A rare and unusual lesion is the congenital granular cell epulis that is present on the mucosa of the alveolar ridge at birth. The occasional presence of odontogenic epithelium among the granular cells has led to the belief that it is an odontogenic tumor, but the odontogenic epithelium is most probably incidental.

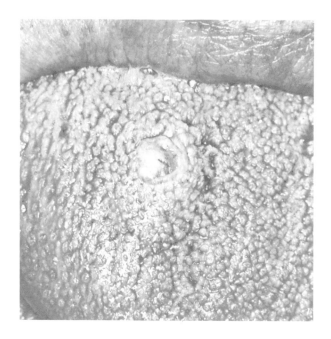

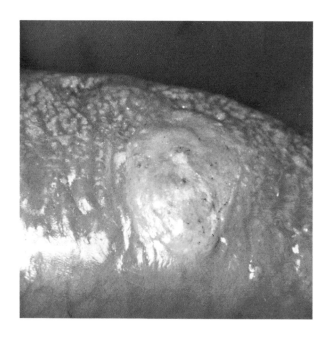

Peripheral ameloblastoma of alveolar ridge.

Peripheral, extraosseus ameloblastoma or ameloblastoma of the soft tissues is a rare tumor that occurs in the soft tissues of the tooth-bearing areas of the mouth. In a study of 180 ameloblastomas 10 percent were of the peripheral type[462]. There is no sex predilection. The mean age has been given as 54 years[462] and 52 years[408] revealing that the peripheral ameloblastoma occurs at a significantly older age than its central (intraosseous) counterpart. In the material from the USA[462] the average duration of the tumor was 15 months. Clinically, the peripheral ameloblastomas are painless, firm in consistency, sessile or pedunculated with an average size of 1.5 cm. Sometimes the tumor has a pink color as in the illustration, which is from an Indian woman. In about 20–30 percent there is a bony depression underneath the lesion. In the American material almost all cases showed a mixture of the typical histologic patterns of ameloblastoma, but the basal cell type was the most common dominant pattern. In one of the reviews of the literature, excluding the gingival basal cell carcinoma, the predominant histologic type was the acanthomatous[203]. In about half the cases, the tumor cells have been in continuity with the surface epithelium. (Courtesy of Dr. D. K. DAFTARY, Bombay, India)

Blue nevus of palate

Pigmented nevi are much less common in the oral mucosa than they are on the skin. The nevi found in the oral mucosa are intramucosal, blue, compound and junctional. Second in frequency among the oral nevi is the blue nevus, which is a benign melanin-producing tumor consisting of melanocytes, generally located deep in connective tissue of the mucosa[83]. The blue nevus cells are more closely related to melanocytes, although they possess some of the characteristics of Schwann cells[337]. An intraoral blue nevus is thought to be present at birth and to undergo no apparent change. An analysis of 32 cases of oral blue nevus has shown that the lesion is seen with equal frequency in men and women[237]. According to the same analysis the oral blue nevus has a predilection for the mucosa of the hard palate, as 72 percent were found in this location. This finding should be compared with the fact that about 50 percent of oral melanomas are located on the hard palate. In this connection it should be stressed that a malignant transformation of an oral blue nevus has never been reported. The picture shows a blue nevus on the hard palate of a 23-year-old man. The histologic examination of the lesion revealed that the blue nevus was associated with an intramucosal nevus, a very rare coincidence.

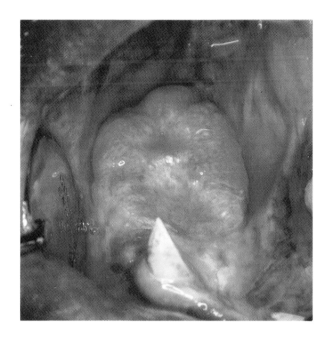

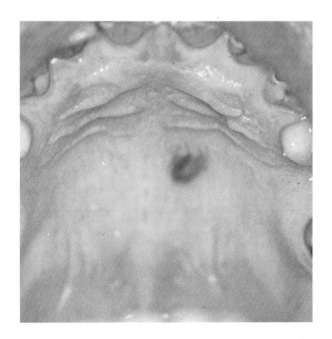

Intramucosal nevus of retromolar area

In one of the largest materials of oral nevi ever published[84] it was found that the intramucosal nevus is the most frequent of all nevi: 55 percent of 107 nevi. The mean size appears to be 0.6 cm. Among 591 intramucosal nevi only three were larger than 1.3 cm. The intramucosal nevus is usually a raised lesion and only 11 percent have been referred to as flat. This feature is of clinical importance in the differential diagnosis from racial pigmentation and other pigmented lesions, such as oral focal melanosis and amalgam tattoo, which are almost always flat lesions[84]. The most common location of the intramucosal nevus is the hard palate, followed by the buccal mucosa[83]. A larger size with a verrucous surface has been reported from Brazil[141]. Most patients with an intramucosal nevus do not have any complaint with regard to the lesion, and most of them are not even aware of its existence. Three-fourths of intramucosal nevi exhibit pigmentation upon clinical examination[84]. The picture illustrates an intramucosal nevus, in a 22-year-old woman, of an unusually large size (6×3 mm). The histologic examination showed the presence of melanin in the nevus cells.

Junctional nevus of palate

The rarest type among the oral nevi is the junctional nevus in which the nevus cells are present in nests or cords in the lower part of the epithelium and/or beneath the epithelium, but still in contact with it[83]. When nevus cells are also present in the deeper part of lamina propria, the nevus becomes of the compound type. Intraorally, the size of junctional nevus is within the range of 0.1 to 1.0 cm and there is no apparent predilection for sex or race[217]. The most frequent intraoral sites for this type of nevus are the palate and buccal mucosa. As the nevus cells in the junctional nevus contain only small amounts of melanin it appears brown, as seen in the illustration opposite. This is from a 4-year-old boy whose mother discovered a palatal brown spot shortly after birth. The spot has not changed in color or size. When the child was 7-years-old the lesion was removed. The histologic diagnosis was junctional nevus. The potential for a junctional nevus to undergo malignant transformation is still unknown because of the paucity of reported cases and the limited follow-up[233]. There is a great similarity between the oral junctional nevi and the melanotic macules, also known as ephelides or lentigo[83].

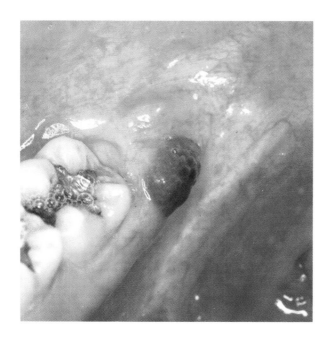

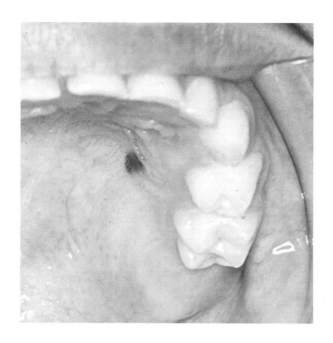

Lentigo maligna of buccal mucosa

Lentigo maligna, also known as lentigo maligna melanoma, Hutchinson's malignant lentigo, precancerous melanosis of Dubreuilh, and acral-lentiginous melanoma, is a premalignant lesion of melanocytes which may progress to malignant melanoma. Lentigo maligna is an uncommon, slowly growing, pigmented freckle, found most frequently on the faces of patients over 50. The pigmented area shows variations in the distribution and intensity of the pigment, which may range from dirty grayish brown to bluish black. Histologically, the lentigo maligna is characterized by an increased pigmentation in the basal cell layer and an increased number both of apparently typical melanocytes and atypical melanocytes. There are only a few reports on intraoral locations of lentigo maligna[75, 456, 466]. They have been located to floor of mouth, buccal mucosa, and palate. Two of these four cases developed into a melanoma with fatal outcome. The illustration shows a lentigo maligna in the buccal mucosa of a 46-year-old man. Two years ago the lesion extended onto the labial mucosa. That area was treated with soft X-rays. Six years after the first examination the pigmentation had disappeared.

Nevus of Ota

Nevus of Ota, also known as nevus fuscocaeruleus ophthalmomaxillaris, or oculodermal melanocytosis, is a unilateral, flat or slightly elevated, blue or gray-brown macula limited to the eye and surrounding skin of the face, innervated by the first and second branches of the trigeminal nerve[382]. The nevus occurs most often in Japanese. There is a predominance of women. The nevus of Ota is usually congenital but may appear in the second decade of life or later. The distribution is usually, but not always, unilateral. The color tones of the nevus fluctuate according to a number of factors, for instance fatigue, menstruation, insomnia, and cloudy weather. In very rare instances a malignant melanoma may develop in the nevus of Ota. The nasal and oral mucosa may be involved. Most often affected in the mouth is the palatal mucosa. Among 177 Japanese with moderate to severe degree of pigmentation 16 percent had pigmentation of the palate[248]. The patient shown opposite is a South Indian woman. Besides the oral manifestation of the nevus of Ota, she also had brown pigmentation of the right sclera and conjunctiva and of the skin of the right cheek (Courtesy of the late Dr. J. ZACHARIAH, Trivandrum, India).

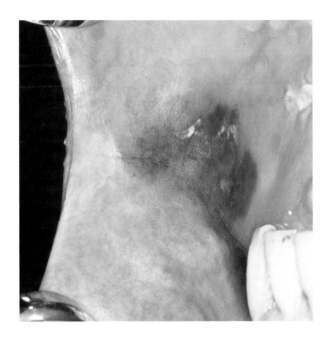

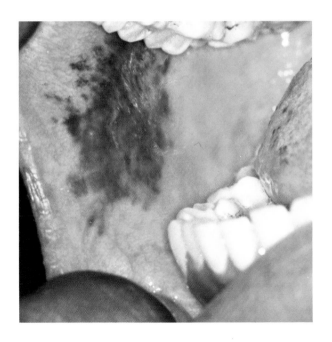

Hemangiopericytoma of palate

Hemangiopericytoma is a benign and largely solid mass of endothelial cells of typical appearance identifiable by the formation of capillaries or other vascular structures in some places. Frequently, this lesion is not clearly separable from capillary hemangioma[168]. Hemangiopericytoma of the oral cavity is rare; so far less than 40 cases have been published[76]. In a review of 33 intraoral hemangiopericytomas eight cases occurred in the tongue, six in the maxilla, five in the mandible, four in the lip, three in the floor of the mouth, three in the buccal mucosa, three in the gingiva and one with multiple lesions in the tongue, soft palate, and lip[76]. There is a wide range in age and a fairly equal distribution according to sex. Clinically, the appearance varies a great deal from a violet-blue tumor to a swelling with normal color. The tumor is characterized by a slow growth, local aggressiveness, and infiltration and frequent recurrences after simple excision. The patient shown here is a 26-year-old man who noticed a swelling 7 weeks before seeking dental help. A biopsy was followed by an extensive bleeding. A surgical excision was followed by a recurrence 3 months later. Histologically the tumor was cell-rich with round or spindle-shaped nuclei and showed an extensive hyperplasia of capillaries[522].

Capillary hemangioma of labial sulcus

After fibromas, angiomas are the most common benign tumors in the oral mucosa. Several investigators have challenged the neoplastic nature of the hemangiomas, which are tumors of the blood vessels. This concept is brought forward by naming the congenital forms of hemangiomas vascular nevi, which are developmental anomalies. Another term is vascular hamartoma, in which excess vessels are present in otherwise normal tissue. A suggestion has been made[518] that the vascular lesions of the oral mucosa be classified into: (1) tumor-like lesions (pyogenic granuloma, p. 210); (2) benign tumors (hamartomas); (3) syndromes with vascular oral lesions (p. 258); (4) malignant tumors. The hemangiomas of the oral mucosa may occur in any area, but the favored site is the lips, especially for the congenital type. The illustration is from a 7-year-old girl, who since birth has had an oral vascular nevus and similar lesions on the left arm and abdomen. The asymptomatic lesion in the maxillary labial sulcus extends slightly onto the alveolar process. A biopsy showed that the nevus consisted of capillaries. When treatment is planned it should be remembered that a number of hemangiomas may show a spontaneous involution.

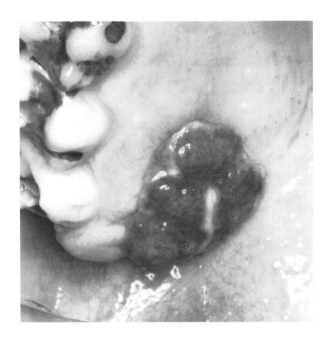

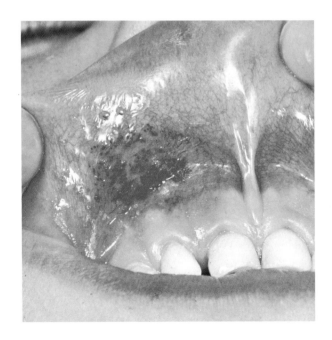

Cavernous hemangioma of tongue

When a hemangioma is composed of large vascular spaces lined by endo-thelial cells it is classified as a cavernous hemangioma. The cavernous hemangioma is either congenital or may appear later in life. It is a common lesion of the oral mucosa and it may be located in any area of the mouth. It is less commonly found in the deeper connective tissue and muscle[518]. The superficial lesions usually have a purple color and a lobulated surface. Occasionally, pulsation is visible. When pressure is exerted on the soft tumor, a blanching appears. The deeper lesions are surrounded or "encap-sulated" by connective tissue and covered with epithelium, so that their color is a light red or pink rather than purple. The cavernous hemangiomas may vary considerably in size; the lingual cavernous hemangioma illus-trated, in a 12-year-old girl, is a rather small lesion. It should be mentioned that cavernous hemangiomas may occur inside the jaws, especially in the mandible, where they should be considered a serious condition. Several cases are reported in which a fatal hemorrhage followed tooth extraction. The occurrence of spurting bleeding or continual oozing of blood from the gingiva may indicate the presence of such a lesion.

Lymphangioma of tongue

Lymphangioma is a benign tumor of lymphatic vessels, although several authors maintain that this lesion should be classified as a hamartoma because a large number of lymphangiomas are found in patients less than 20 years of age. By far the majority of the lymphangiomas are located on the tongue, especially on the dorsum anteriorly. Lymphangiomas also may be found on the lips and the buccal mucosa, in the latter location occasionally extending to the orbital area. The tumor may be unilateral, but most often it is bilateral. Lymphangiomas exhibit a marked variation with regard to size, ranging from pin-head size lesions to extensive infiltra-tion of the entire tongue and surrounding structures. The affected surface of the tongue is characterized by irregular nodules, sometimes even papil-lary projections, which are gray, pink, or yellow-brown, depending on the amount of erythrocytes in the lymph fluid. The patient shown here is a 17-year-old girl who had an exophytic type of a lymphangioma on the dorsum of the tongue, a typical location for this tumor.

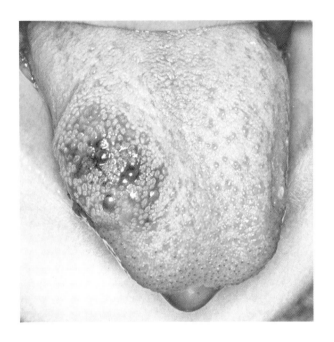

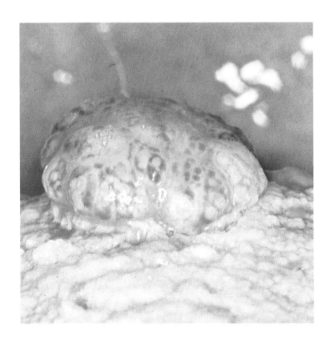

Cystic hygroma

When located on the tongue, the lymphangioma will in most cases cause macroglossia. Some investigators consider a diffuse lymphangioma to be the most common cause of macroglossia[464]. This is especially apparent in the cervical cystic hygroma (lymphangioma cavernosum), which is an infiltrating lymphangioma involving the neck and seen in children at birth. The lymphangiomatous tissue may extend from the tongue and sublingual area through the submandibular region upward into the cheek and the parotid region and downward into the neck, sometimes causing an enormous swelling. The process may be either unilateral or bilateral. The enlarged tongue will protrude outside the oral cavity, so that its surface becomes dry and sometimes ulcerated. The diffuse swelling of the tongue and floor of the mouth will give rise to obstruction of the upper respiratory and alimentary passages, occasionally necessitating tracheotomy. Speech is also gravely impaired and development of the jaw may be irregular[179]. A rather mild case of cystic hygroma in a 2½-year-old boy is illustrated opposite. Besides the macroglossia, the boy also suffered from a swelling in the floor of the mouth caused by the cystic hygroma.

Neurofibromatosis

Generalized multiple neurofibromatosis (Recklinghausen's neurofibromatosis) is characterized by pigmentation of the skin and cutaneous and subcutaneous neurofibromas. Neurofibromatosis is considered to be a malformation, and about 40 percent of the cases show hereditary transmission. There is a controversy as to the exact identity of the lesion tissue, which by some is considered to be nerve tissue proper and by others to be fibroblastic and of endoneural and perineural origin. The skin tumors, which vary greatly in size, may be present at birth or appear during childhood or even later. Oral manifestations in neurofibromatosis comprise six different types including macroglossia, hyperplasia of lingual papillae and/or isolated or multiple superficial tumors[32]. The oral changes may resemble soft fibromas or papillomas. The patient shown here is a 20-year-old woman with neurofibromatosis also associated with café-au-lait spots on the skin. When found in the mouth the disease may extend into the floor of the mouth and the submandibular area, indicating that not only the lingual, but also the hypoglossal and glossopharyngeal nerves may be involved[448-]

124

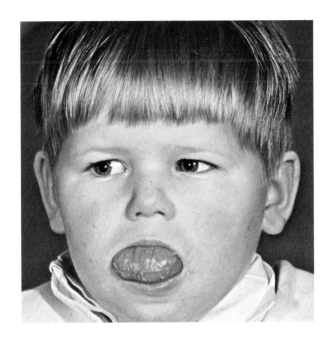

NEOPLASMS OF UNCERTAIN BEHAVIOR OF NERVOUS SYSTEM

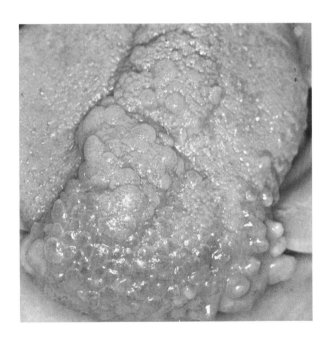

Multiple mucosal neuroma syndrome

Among the familial syndromes of Multiple Endocrine Neoplasia (MEN) one type[16] is characterized by mucosal neuromas, pheochromocytoma, and medullary thyroid carcinoma[215]. Additional features are a marfanoid appearance and bumpy lips. In 1975 there were 41 cases reported in the literature[298] of the syndrome, thought to be one of hyperplasia and/or neoplasia or neural crest derivation and fitting into a scheme of neuroendocrine syndromes. A majority of the patients with the syndrome have a characteristic facial appearance with diffusely enlarged lips, some show prognathism and have acromegalic facial appearance. So far, mucosal neuromas have been present in all the reported cases of the syndrome; oral neuromas in 90 percent[278]. The tongue is affected in 92 percent of the patients with oral involvement. The illustration shows typical neuromas along the margin of the tongue in a 12-year-old boy with the syndrome. The lips are the seat of neuromas in 78 percent, whereas the remaining parts of the oral mucosa only rarely are affected by neuromas. Histologically, the neuromas appear as unencapsulated masses of convoluted nerves representing hypertrophy of axons similar to the changes found in amputation neuromas.

ENDOCRINE, NUTRITIONAL, AND METABOLIC DISEASES

Athyroidism

The term hypothyroidism is used to signify all forms of hypofunction of the thyroid gland. Athyroidism is the type of hypothyroidism in which functioning thyroid tissue cannot be demonstrated. Such a condition is illustrated here in a 6-month-old girl, where scanning with ^{131}I revealed total absence of functioning thyroid tissue. The child was admitted to the hospital because of the macroglossia. This sign may be present in hypothyroidism, and can give rise to difficulties in eating and speaking. Often this enlargement of the tongue is so pronounced that there is a constant protrusion. The macroglossia[598] is caused by a mucoproteinous infiltration, which also may affect the lips. The oral mucosa tends to be dry. After adequate treatment the macroglossia will disappear. In hypothyroidism the head is large in comparison to the body, and closure of the fontanels is considerably delayed. The eruption of teeth is retarded in children with hypothyroidism, although bone development is less retarded. There is also a high frequency of enamel hypoplasia among hypothyroid children[11].

126

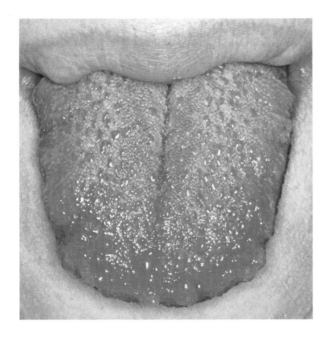

Disorders of Thyroid Gland

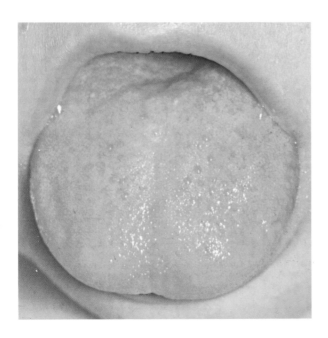

Diabetes mellitus

Diabetes mellitus has a prevalence of 0.5 to 1.7 percent in the general population. It is a chronic disease characterized by an increase of glucose in the blood and the excretion of glucose in the urine; its severity depends on the deficient formation of insulin secreted by the β-cells of the islets of Langerhans of the pancreas. The characteristic symptoms are general weakness, weight loss, increased thirst, and polyuria. In diabetes mellitus there is a reduced resistance to infection, notably with *Candida albicans*. Early indications of diabetes mellitus may consist of a feeling of dryness and burning of the tongue and gingival tenderness. Lingual central papillary atrophy has been found in 17 percent of diabetics, and in 43 percent of these *Candida*-hyphae were found[178]. In uncontrolled diabetics the gingiva may be hypertrophic, or may show irregular proliferations, as in the 18-year-old girl shown here. Other periodontal manifestations are easy gingival bleeding, violaceous gingival hue, pocket formation in children, and increased tooth mobility. In a study of diabetic children with poor metabolic control, the Gingival Index scores were higher than among the non-diabetics, while no such tendency was seen in diabetics with good metabolic control[208].

Acromegaly

An overactivity of the pituitary gland leading to an overproduction of the growth hormone will cause gigantism in children and acromegaly in adults. The etiology of the hypersecretion is usually an eosinophilic adenoma of the pituitary gland. Acromegaly is associated with characteristic clinical findings dominated by overgrowth of the terminal bones, especially of the hands and feet, and presence of massive frontal bosses. The ears, nose, and lips are enlarged, which contributes to the typical acromegalic facial expression characterized by coarseness. The tongue is enlarged in 50 percent. The macroglossia is due primarily to an increased diameter of the muscle fibers; but hyperplasia of epithelium and connective tissue also contribute to the enlargement[598]. The mandibular growth centers are stimulated, especially the condyle, which causes a mesial sliding of the bite, leading to a prominence of the chin. The width of the mandible is also increased, probably because of the enlarged tongue, which is a constant feature in acromegaly[571]. The macroglossia, occasionally marked by indentations, will give rise also to spacing and labial tilting of the teeth. The patient shown here is a 58-year-old woman with a 5-year-old acromegaly which had caused a marked enlargement of the tongue.

128

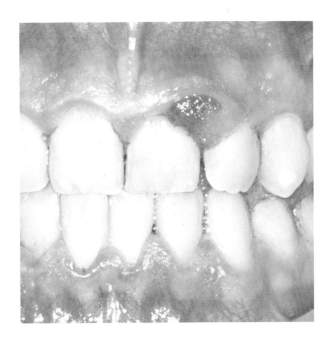

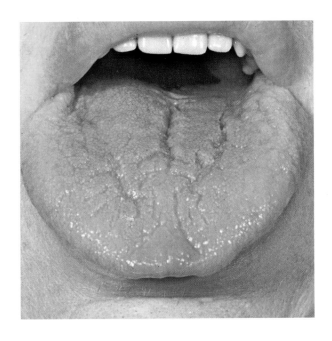

Hypoadrenocorticism

Hypoadrenocorticism, also known as Addison's disease, is due to an adrenal cortical hypofunction which may be the result of idiopathic atrophy or a loss of function caused by other diseases, especially tuberculosis, amyloidosis, or tumors. Clinically, the disease is characterized mainly by weakness, anorexia, weight loss, hypotension, nausea, and vomiting. In addition, often as an early sign, the patients exhibit a bronze-like pigmentation of the skin, especially in pressure points and at the palmar creases; the oral mucosa also becomes hyperpigmented. The pigmentation is supposedly due to an increased production of the melanocyte-stimulating hormone. The oral pigmentation varies in intensity and in color. It may be pale brown, dirty grayish, or even blackish. Although the oral pigmentation may be found in any area of the mouth, the buccal mucosa is the most frequent site, as in the patient shown here, a 38-year-old man who had been treated for Addison's disease for the past 20 years. The picture shows his right buccal mucosa, but he also has pigmented areas on the lower lip and the soft palate. Some authors maintain that the oral pigmentation disappears following therapy; others believe that the increased melanin deposit is not influenced by the treatment.

Protein malnutrition (kwashiorkor)

Protein deficiency is rather common in tropical countries. Children on a diet low in protein and high in calories may develop kwashiorkor (a West African word meaning "disease occurring in a young child displaced from his mother by a subsequent pregnancy"), although kwashiorkor is never exclusively dietary in etiology. Infective, psychologic, cultural, and other conditioning factors are also contributory[278]. The clinical signs of kwashiorkor are growth retardation, edema of the extremities, muscle wasting with retention of some subcutaneous fat, swelling of the abdomen, sparseness and dyspigmentation of the hair, and psychomotor change. A study[419] among children with kwashiorkor in Bangalore in South India showed more cases of acute necrotizing gingivitis, candidiasis, atrophy of tongue papillae, coated tongue, and angular cheilosis than among healthy children in a control group. Furthermore, the Periodontal Index and the PMA Index showed significantly higher values in the kwashiorkor group. The 6-year-old boy shown here is from that study. The child exhibitis sparsity of hair, dry skin, and angular cheilosis. In evaluating the effect of kwashiorkor, it should be remembered that vitamin deficiencies, especially vitamin A deficiency, may occur simultaneously with kwashiorkor.

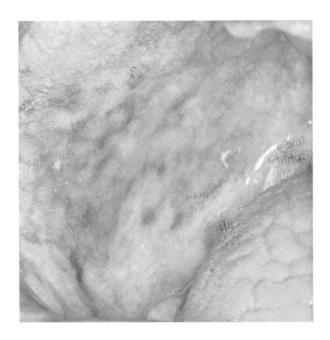

NUTRITIONAL DEFICIENCIES

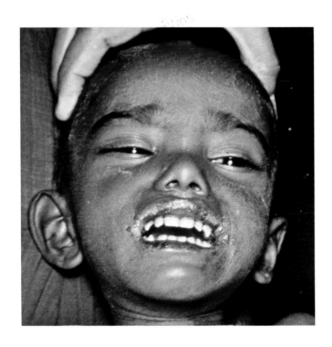

Niacin deficiency

Niacin or nicotinic acid is one of the vitamins belonging to the vitamin B complex. A deficiency of this vitamin causes development of pellagra. The disease has been eradicated in most parts of the world, but is still endemic in some areas where green vegetables and meats are scarce. It is seen also in alcoholics. Prodromal symptoms of pellagra are loss of appetite and weight, indigestion, diarrhea, abdominal pain, and burning sensations in various parts of the body. Later dermatitis of sun-exposed areas develops. The nervous system also becomes involved. Early in the course of pellegra oral changes appear in the form of glossitis, stomatitis, and gingivitis, which may constitute the presenting complaint[397]. The most characteristic changes are observed on the tongue. In the early stages only the tip and margins of the tongue are swollen and red. In the advanced and severe cases the tongue loses all the papillae and the reddening becomes intense, as in the illustration, which is of a 31-year-old Brazilian woman. In this stage the tongue may become so swollen that indentations from the teeth are found along the borders of the tongue. At the same time the tongue is extremely sensitive. The remaining oral mucosa becomes reddened and ulcerated. (Courtesy of Dr. Bopp, Porto Alegre, Brazil).

Ascorbic acid deficiency

Ascorbic acid, or vitamin C, is necessary for the hydroxylation of proline in collagen synthesis as it occurs in the intercellular substance of connective tissue, bone, and dentin. Deficiency in ascorbic acid may lead to the clinical condition, scurvy, known for centuries, characterized by weakness and hemorrages in the skin, muscles, joints, and alimentary tract. The cutaneous hemorrhages may occur as petechiae or ecchymoses, and are most marked on the legs and buttocks. Usually, the gingiva in both jaws are markedly swollen and spongy and demonstrate several areas of mucosal bleeding, as in the 55-year-old woman shown here, who was admitted to the hospital because of spontaneous bleeding from the gingiva. Parts of the marginal gingiva and interdental papillae are covered by fibrin. A clinical examination revealed a number of changes typical of scurvy. For several years her diet had consisted of bread, meat and pastries, with no vegetables. Only rarely do case reports on scurvy presenting oral symptoms appear in the literature[175, 556]. However, recently a 9-year-old American girl was found to have scurvy with severe gingival erosions. A dietary history disclosed that she consumed only one kind of sandwich and beverage and took no other foods[162].

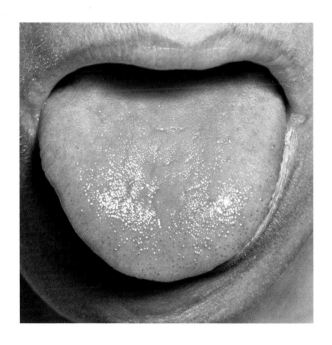

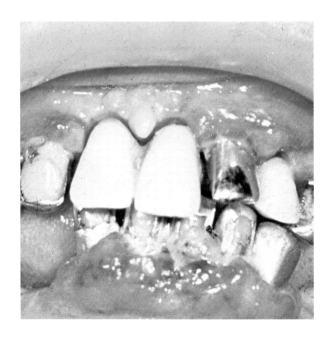

133

Urbach-Wiethe disease

The Urbach-Wiethe disease (UWD), also called lipoglycoproteinosis, or lipoid proteinosis or hyalinosis cutis et mucosae, is a rare recessively inherited disorder of unknown etiology characterized by visible lesions in the skin and in the mucous membranes of the mouth, pharynx and larynx[55]. Histologically, the connective tissue contains extracellular deposits of a hyaline-like material which contains glycoproteins and small lipid droplets. The most striking symptom is hoarseness, usually present since early childhood, caused by deposits in the vocal cords. In a material of 27 patients with UWD from Northern Sweden oral changes were found in all the patients[256]. The areas most frequently affected were the labial mucosa, the posterior part of the tongue, the lingual frenulum, and the palate. In teenage patients granular lesions of the labial mucosa and palate were observed. With increasing age, the affected mucosa seems to become more pale in color and pitted in structure. The lingual frenulum becomes short, indurated and thick, as is seen in the 51-year-old man shown opposite[256]. In older patients the mucosal changes were more indurated, giving the mucosa a scarred, firm and glossy appearance. (Courtesy of Dr. A. BERGENHOLTZ, Umeå, Sweden).

Macroglobulinemia

Macroglobulinemia, also called macroglobulinemia of Waldenström, is a relatively rare, chronic, idiopathic, probably neoplastic disturbance of the reticuloendothelial system resulting in the production of large globulin molecules and a typical clinical picture. The outcome is usually fatal, although the course may be protracted. The syndrome occurs most often between the ages of 50 and 70. Initial symptoms, such as weakness, general malaise, dyspnea, and loss of appetite and weight, are followed by purpura and bleeding from eyes, mouth, nose, and from other mucous membranes. The lymph nodes often are swollen, the spleen and liver are increased in size, and neurologic symptoms may be present. Most patients suffer from anemia. Gingival bleeding, due to a concurrent hemorrhagic diathesis, is an outstanding feature, and the patients may awaken in the morning with their mouths full of blood[580]. Persistent hemorrhage after tooth extraction has been reported. Petechiae and ecchymoses of the oral mucosa are seen in the 77-year-old woman pictured here, who also suffered from bleeding from the vermilion border. Some investigators have reported peculiar and painful ulcerations of the oral mucosa[202], and swelling of the submandibular lymph nodes as initial symptoms of macroglobulinemia.

134

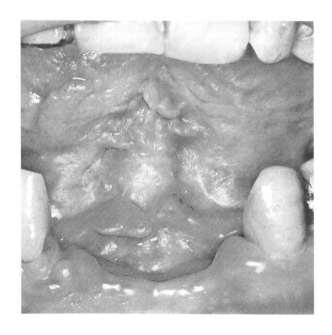

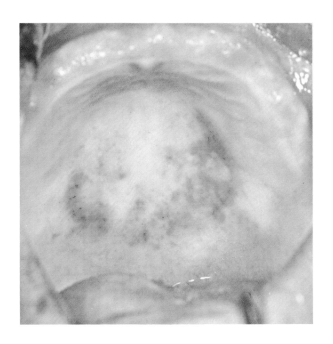

Mucoviscoidosis

Mucoviscoidosis (syn. cystic fibrosis of pancreas, fibrocystic disease) is a generalized, inherited disease of unknown etiology associated with dysfunction of all exocrine glands. The incidence of the disease is 1 per 2,000 live births. The basic metabolic defect is not known. The abnormal secretions which occur in mucoviscoidosis have been recognized as the basic pathologic lesion which results in bronchial and pancreatic obstruction. The mean p_H and buffering capacity of stimulated saliva is higher than in normal controls and the caries experience less than that of controls[300]. The submandibular saliva contains about 65 percent more lipids/100 ml than that of controls[525]. The oral manifestations consist primarily of changes due to the inspissated mucus produced by the salivary glands. The labial mucosa becomes dry and swollen, which is illustrated opposite in a 6-year-old boy, who suffers from mucoviscoidosis. In a material of 22 lip biopsies from children with the disease 72 percent showed changes in the form of duct dilatation, flattening of ductal epithelium, inspissated eosinophilic material in ducts and acini and, in advanced cases, atrophy of acini and fibrosis[564]. It was concluded that a lip biopsy may confirm the diagnosis of mucoviscoidosis in most cases.

Amyloidosis

Amyloidosis is a rare disorder characterized by accumulation of amyloid, a fibrillar protein of unknown composition, in various tissues of the body. Amyloid is demonstrated by means of special stains such as congo red, metachromatic dyes, and fluorochromic dyes, such as thioflavin T. Amyloid probably is produced in the reticuloendothelial cells and deposited intercellularly in the ground substance. In primary amyloidosis, amyloid is deposited around blood vessels, in skin, heart, kidney, liver, gastrointestinal tract, larynx and trachea. The prognosis of amyloidosis is grave; the life expectancy after the onset of symptoms is approximately 3 years. An enlarged tongue is one of the most frequent features of primary amyloidosis causing difficulties in chewing, swallowing, or talking. The speech difficulties may also be due to paresis of the vocal cords resulting from deposits of amyloid in the upper third of the larynx[570]. The patient seen here is a 71-year-old woman who had suffered from difficulties in swallowing due to an enlarged tongue. She is unusual in that the amyloid deposits have caused a tumor-like enlargement of the left side of the tongue. The mucosal folds close to the labial commissures are characteristic for oral manifestations of amyloidosis.

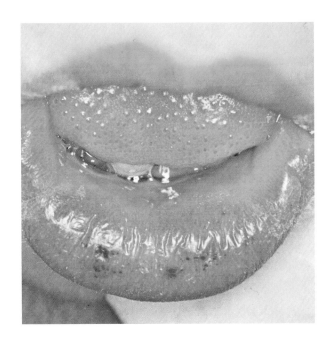

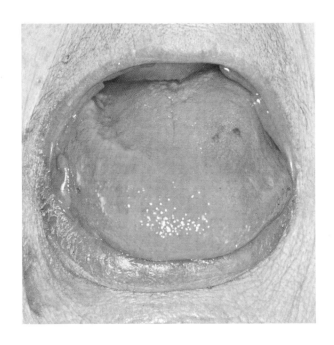

Amyloidosis

The clinical manifestations of primary amyloidosis depend upon which organ or organs have been the site of deposition of amyloid. Muscle involvement may lead to a macroglossia (see p. 136) as the initial symptom. Purpuric spots, caused by hemorrhage resulting from amyloid deposits in the blood vessels, may be seen on the skin and mucous membranes. The illustration shows ecchymoses in the buccal mucosa of a 63-year-old man with primary amyloidosis. Some of the areas of submucosal bleeding have become the site of hyperkeratotic excrescences, a feature which is rarely reported in the literature[531]. The patient had similar lesions on the tongue, labial mucosa, and in the floor of the mouth. He died from his disease 6 months after the oral examination. Besides the primary amyloidosis there are three other types: (1) secondary, associated with chronic infection or chronic inflammation, (2) amyloid associated with multiple myeloma, and (3) hereditary. In the second edition of this Atlas there was an illustration of a tongue which was the seat of macroglossia caused by deposits of amyloid as a result of a myeloma. Seven to 10 percent of patients with multiple myeloma have associated amyloidosis[308].

Hypercarotinemia

When large amounts of carotene-containing foods (mainly carrots, oranges, sweet potatoes and egg yolks) are ingested, the blood plasma may contain a high enough concentration of pigment to impart a yellowish color to the skin, especially the palms of the hands, behind the ears, and the nasolabial folds. Also the oral mucosa may be affected, especially the palate, with a yellow to orange pigmentation. The illustration opposite shows a marked yellow color of the soft palate in a 54-year-old woman who suffered from carotinemia. She had been eating substantial amounts of carrots daily causing a slightly yellowish color in her face. Whereas the blood value for vitamin A was normal, there was an increase in the value for carotene. The patient was asked to reduce her consumption of carrots. Four months later the blood carotene value had returned to normal, but the oral pigmentation remained unchanged. Carotinemia should be distinguished from jaundice, which also is associated with a yellow color of the skin. Whereas the jaundice also causes a yellow color of the sclera, carotinemia does not involve the sclera. The diagnosis of carotinemia is made by laboratory findings of serum carotene.

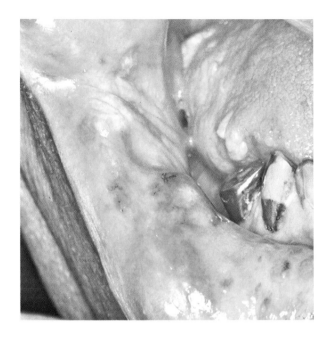

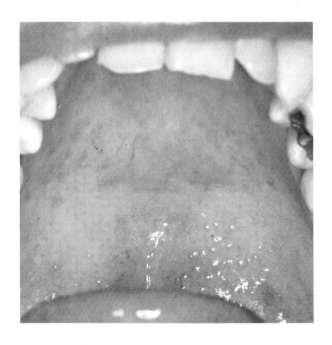

Eosinophilic granuloma of bone

Eosinophilic granuloma of bone (localized histiocytosis) is one of the three entities contained in the concept of histiocytosis X[235]. The other two are Hand-Schüller-Christian disease (chronic disseminated histiocytosis) and Letterer-Siwe disease (acute disseminated histiocytosis). The underlying common denominator is the development of granulomatous lesions with histiocytic proliferation[127]. In the eosinophilic bone granuloma the lesion may occur in the jawbone and overlying soft tissues of the oral cavity, so that the differential diagnosis between eosinophilic granuloma and other oral mucosal diseases may become a problem. The picture opposite illustrates such a case. It is of a 15-year-old boy, who was referred for multiple ulcerations of the oral mucosa apparently originating from the gingiva. The illustration shows the characteristic appearance in one of the locations palatal to the maxillary right first and second molars. Mesial to a half-erupted mandibular third molar there was a radiolucent zone. Biopsies from the affected regions showed the characteristic features of an eosinophilic granuloma. Lesions of the gingiva have also been described in patients with histiocytosis X[216].

Chronic granulomatous disease

Chronic granulomatous disease (CGD), first described as an entity in 1957, is an inherited disorder characterized by an inability of the polymorphonuclear leukocytes (PMN) to kill ingested bacteria. Underlying the bactericidal defect is an inability of the patient's PMN to convert oxygen into metabolites that reduce nitroblue tetrazolium dye[284]. Previously, the disease was called fatal granulomatous disease of childhood. Most patients with CGD exhibit an x-linked mode of inheritance, with occasional cases transmitted by an autosomal recessive gene[284]. The male:female ratio is 6:1. The inability of the leukocytes to kill bacteria results in a clinical picture characterized by a wide spectrum of infections including marked lymphadenopathy, often with suppuration, pneumonitis, dermatitis, hepatomegaly, splenomegaly, osteomyelitis, etc. Oral manifestations are found in 18 percent of patients with CGD[284]. The oral changes reported have been recurrent ulcerative stomatitis, parallel folds of hyperplastic tissue and aphthous-like ulcerations[9, 613]. The picture is of a 10-year-old boy, who has suffered from recurrent oral ulcerations in the last 7–8 years. Aphthous-like ulcerations are present on the labial and buccal mucosa and gingiva.

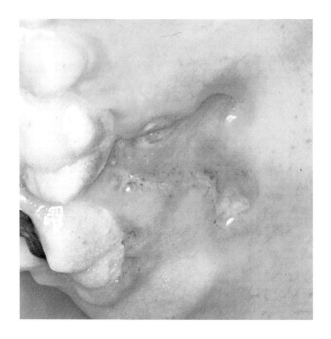

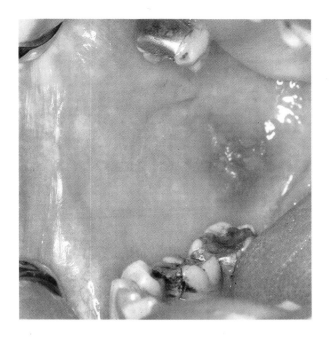

Chronic granulomatous disease

The illustration opposite is from the mouth of the mother of the boy shown on the preceding page. The patient is 39 years old; she has suffered from oral ulcerations for 15 years, with one attack every 3 month always located to the left buccal mucosa. She also suffers from hidradenitis and hand eczema and acute glomerulonephritis. The patient is a carrier of x-linked CGD. She shows a decreased intracellular killing of *Staph. aureus* by leukocytes in vitro. In a material of 23 mothers with children having CGD, 83 percent had the intermediate defect of function of leukocytes that identifies the heterozygous carrier state[284]. The function of individual leukocytes can be examined by determining their ability to reduce nitro-blue tetrazolium dye after stimulation by phagocytosis or contact with endotoxin. However, most carriers are free of undue infections, but skin diseases including discoid lupus erythematosus and recurrent aphthous stomatitis have been reported. In a series of nine carriers of x-linked CGD, three had discoid lupus erythematosus-like skin lesions which histologically were consistent with DLE. Four had experienced photosensitivity in childhood and seven had recurrent aphthous-like stomatitis which should be distinguished from the recurrent aphthous ulcerations seen in otherwise healthy individuals[72].

Acquired immunodeficiency syndrome – candidiasis

For the sake of surveillance for AIDS, two criteria should be met: (1) the presence of a reliably diagnosed disease at least moderately predictive of cellular immune deficiency, and (2) the absence of an underlying cause for the immune deficiency or of any defined cause for reduced resistance to disease[154]. Up to 1984, 3000 cases had been reported in the USA. Of these 71 percent were homosexual or bisexual men, or i.v. drug users, and 4.5 percent were individuals of Haitian origin, 0.6 percent were hemophilics and 6.3 percent "others"[154]. After a period of 1 to 6 months, non-specific illness of variable severity comprising weight loss, fever, night sweating and malaise occurs. Then opportunistic infections develop, such as candidiasis, Pneumocystis carinii, pneumonia, cytomegalic virus, and herpes simplex infections. In a material from San Francisco of 53 homosexuals with Kaposi's sarcoma, 57 percent had oral candidiasis[340]. The illustration is of a 29-year-old man who has had an oral candidiasis as part of his AIDS for months. In another material of homosexual men from San Francisco a hairy type of leukoplakia on the tongue has been demonstrated. This leukoplakia may be associated with both papillomavirus and a herpes-type virus[221].

142

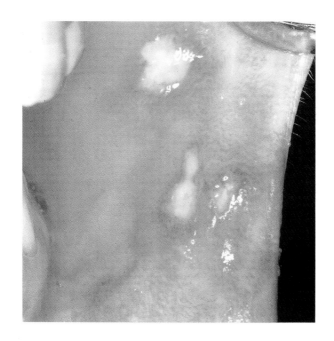

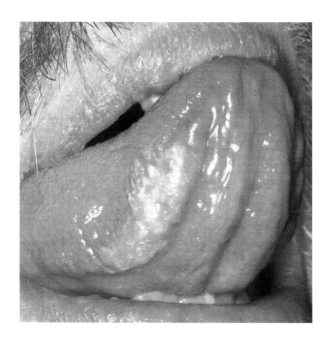

Acquired immunodeficiency syndrome – Kaposi's sarcoma

The impaired immune surveillance present in AIDS patients often leads to the development of Kaposi's sarcoma. However, the immune deficiency in AIDS patients may also be associated with other malignancies, including squamous cell carcinoma of the oral cavity. About 35 percent of all USA patients with AIDS develop Kaposi's sarcoma. In a material of 53 homosexual men with Kaposi's sarcoma from San Francisco, 27 (51 percent) had oral manifestations of the sarcoma[340]. Among the 27 patients with oral manifestations, 89 percent had lesions in the palate, as in the 34-year-old homosexual Danish man illustrated opposite. He has lived in the USA for 6 years and has had syphilis and hepatitis. He was referred to a skin department with cutaneous changes. A biopsy revealed Kaposi's sarcoma. Later lesions appeared in the palate. The spreading of AIDS in homosexual communities quickly gave rise to a strong suspicion of an infectious agent, likely to be a virus. Recent findings from France and the USA have supported the hypothesis that AIDS is caused by a human T-lymphotropic virus (HTLV). The one identified in the USA has been called HTLV-III and the French one LAV (lymphadenopathy-associated virus)[154]. (By courtesy of Dr. I. LORENZEN, Hvidovre, Denmark)

DISEASES OF THE BLOOD AND BLOOD-FORMING ORGANS

Iron deficiency anemia

Iron deficiency anemia may be caused by a chronic blood loss, insufficient iron intake, or defective iron absorption. Women are affected more often than men; the favored age is the 3rd or 4th decade. The anemic patient complains of weakness and dyspnea on exertion; clinically the skin is pale and the nails tend to crack and split. Oral changes are seen quite often. In a sample of 371 British patients, 39 percent had an atrophy of the tongue papillae and 14 percent had an angular cheilosis (rhagades)[61]. In a sample of 110 anemic Sri Lankan women, 37 percent had either partial or total atrophic changes of the tongue, but only 5 percent had angular cheilosis[445]. In an Indian study[137] there was a definite increase in the prevalence of atrophic glossitis with a progressive increase of severity of anemia. Atrophic changes on the dorsum of the tongue usually appear first at the tip and lateral borders, with loss of filiform papillae. In extreme cases the whole dorsum appears smooth and glazed. The tongue, which may be very painful, is either pale or fiery red. The remaining oral mucosa may show pallor. The patient seen here is a 55-year-old woman with marked papillary atrophy, erythema, and angular cheilosis[137].

144

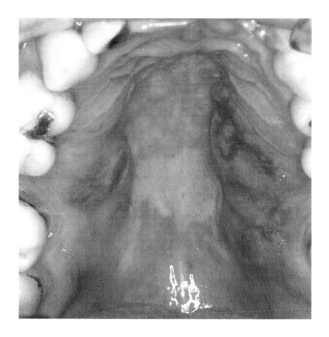

IRON DEFICIENCY ANEMIA

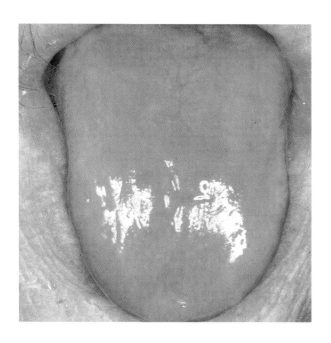

Sideropenic dysphagia

Sideropenic dysphagia[579] is also known as Paterson-Brown Kelly syndrome or Plummer-Vinson syndrome. The condition is found almost exclusively in middle-aged women, and there is often a history of fatigability, anemia, and difficulty in swallowing. Iron deficiency is the primary cause of the syndrome, with dietary deficiencies of vitamins and animal proteins playing an additional role. Patients with sideropenic dysphagia are usually pale, with a characteristic asthenic appearance. The nails are brittle and spoon-shaped (koilonychia). Dysphagia is the outstanding symptom and is attributed to the formation of web in the esophagus. A hypochromic, microcytic anemia is present in the majority of the patients. The vermilion border of the lips is very thin, and there is often angular cheilosis. The width of the mouth is narrowed, and the oral mucosa is pale and atrophic. In 50 to 70 percent of patients there is an atrophy of the tongue papillae[285], and leukoplakia has been reported in a number of cases. The oral changes may be conceived as a precancerous condition, and multiple oral carcinomas sometimes develop in these patients, as in the 72-year-old woman shown here, who developed five independent oral carcinomas in the course of 6 years.

Pernicious anemia

Pernicious anemia, which has a prevalence of about 0.5 percent in the Danish population, usually is seen after the third decade with about equal frequency in both sexes, and with a tendency towards a familial occurrence. Pernicious anemia is caused by a lack of vitamin B_{12}, which is due to a deficiency of the "intrinsic factor" responsible for the resorption of vitamin B_{12} and secreted by certain parts of the stomach. There is a megaloblastic, macrocytic anemia and a failure to secrete free hydrochloric acid after maximal stimulation with histamine. It has been suggested that pernicious anemia is an autoimmune disorder, as autoantibodies to the gastric parietal cells are often found in patients with pernicious anemia. The patients suffer from a general weakness, loss of appetite and weight, dizziness, and numbness or tingling of the extremities. Clinically, the skin has a yellowish tinge, and the hair may be gray. Oral symptoms are often present in the form of (1) paresthesia of the tongue; (2) a burning or itching sensation from the oral mucous membrane; (3) a disturbance in taste; (4) intolerance to dentures; (5) occasional dryness of the mouth.

IRON DEFICIENCY ANEMIA

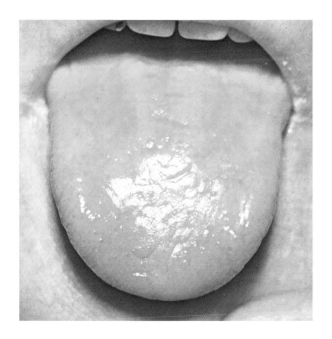

OTHER DEFICIENCY ANEMIA

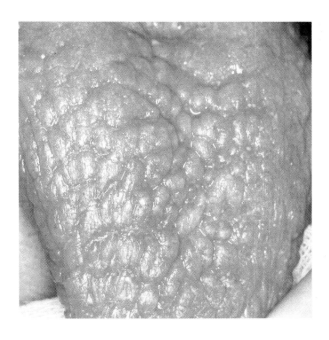

Pernicious anemia

A clinical examination of the oral mucous membrane in patients with pernicious anemia will, in 50 to 60 percent of the cases, reveal changes consisting primarily in loss of the filiform and fungiform papillae, as seen in the 79-year-old woman above. In advanced cases the dorsum of the tongue presents a completely atrophic, smooth, fiery red surface, which may be the site of small erosions. The tongue appears flabby because the normal muscle tonus is reduced. In contrast to the lingual findings in iron deficiency anemia, the tongue in pernicious anemia may show a lobulation, as seen in the illustration. This phenomenon may be secondary to a decrease in saliva production which sometimes is found in these patients[253]. The lobulation is similar to the findings in Sjögren's syndrome (p. 262). The lingual changes in pernicious anemia often are so characteristic that a tentative diagnosis can be made. In some cases subjective tongue symptoms are not associated with clinical changes and may therefore be mistaken for a glossodynia. The oral mucosa in patients with pernicious anemia may exhibit an irregular red erythema[220] as seen in the 46-year-old woman (opposite). Oral aphthous ulcerations occasionally are present in cases of pernicious anemia.

Thrombasthenia

Hemorrhagic diathesis due to disorders of thrombocytes occurs when the number of thrombocytes is reduced and when the thrombocytes fail to function normally. Among the latter disorders is thrombasthenia, which is a defective thrombocyte aggregation. The disease, often called Glanzmann's thrombasthenia, has an autosomal recessive inheritance. The principal finding is a normal release reaction with collagen and thrombin, but the released adenosine diphosphate (ADP) fails to induce thrombocyte aggregation. The released ADP does, however, stimulate the change in thrombocyte shape. It seems, therefore, that receptors for ADP, collagen, and thrombin are present on the thrombocyte membranes but that these membranes lack an essential component for normal aggregation[541]. The patient shown here is an 8-year-old boy who had a thrombasthenia diagnosed at the age of 2 years. Since that time there have been episodes of epistaxis and he had had two extractions done under hospitalization where the bleeding was controlled by thrombocyte-enriched plasma and EACA (epsilon-amino-capronic acid). In connection with an herpetic gingivostomatitis at the age of 8 years the boy had bleedings from his gingiva, which is the seat of ecchymoses as seen in the illustration[409].

148

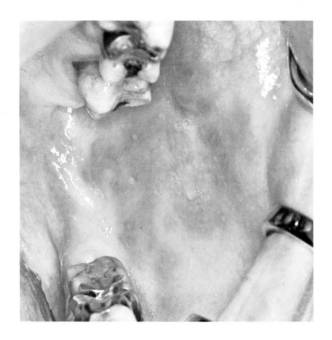

PURPURA AND OTHER HEMORRHAGIC CONDITIONS

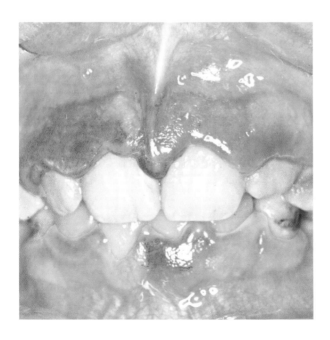

Thrombocytopenia

Thrombocytopenia is a marked decrease in the number of blood platelets. The decrease may be without known cause: idiopathic (essential) thrombocytopenic purpura, or secondary (symptomatic) as a result of a variety of conditions such as infections, malignant tumors, leukemia, lupus erythematosus, and drug hypersensitivity[45]. Purpura, which refers to the purple-colored petechiae or ecchymoses seen on the skin and mucous membranes, may be a sign in several types of hemorrhagic diatheses. Often gingival bleeding may be the first manifestation of the disease. The patient seen here is a 35-year-old woman, previously healthy, who 8 days after a Caesarian section developed a severe hemorrhagic diathesis. The first symptoms were a profuse gingival bleeding and numerous petechiae and ecchymoses in all parts of the oral mucosa. Laboratory findings showed a decrease in the number of thrombocytes and a prolonged bleeding time. It cannot be excluded that the disease may have been caused by a hypersensitivity to barbiturates or penicillin. A grave thrombocytopenia with marked oral ecchymoses has been reported as the result of an immunologic response to the quinine used to "cut" heroin[307].

Malignant neutropenia

Malignant neutropenia is often called agranulocytosis, but the former term is preferred because there are other types of agranulocytosis than the malignant, acute form. Malignant neutropenia may be idiopathic, but is more often a complication of acute leukemia or, in most cases, induced by drugs. A number of drugs may cause malignant neutropenia, especially amidopyrine, chloramphenicol, and the thiouracil group of antithyroid drugs. The onset of the disease is sudden, with a rapid rise in temperature, sore throat, chills, sweating, headache, and prostration. Twelve to 24 hours after these symptoms arise, infective lesions appear, most prominently in the mouth and throat. In severe cases, death occurs, usually caused by pneumonia, a few days after the first symptoms. The oral lesions in malignant neutropenia are necrotizing ulcerations, which often have a punched-out appearance. They are covered by fibrin, but do not have an erythematous halo. In some cases the alveolar bone may become exposed[547]. The lip lesion illustrated is from a 37-year-old woman who developed a malignant neutropenia in relation to treatment with thimazol (Thycapsol). A similar lesion was found in the buccal mucosa, but no acute gingivitis was observed.

150

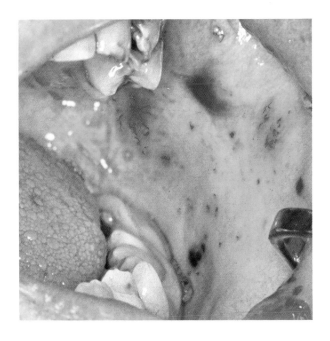

DISEASES OF WHITE BLOOD CELLS

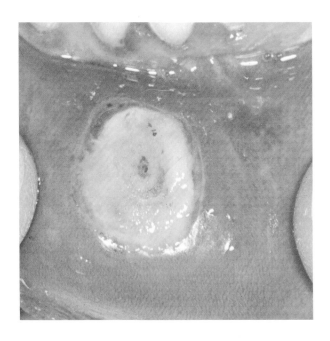

Cyclic neutropenia

In 1949, it was reported that some cases of neutropenia exhibit a cyclic or periodic course. The cyclic neutropenia is characterized by a periodic disappearance of circulating neutrophils. These cells disappear from or are markedly reduced in the peripheral blood at intervals of approximately 3 weeks. After a 5- to 8-day period the neutrophils increase in number, but are always somewhat sparser than normal. The neutropenic phase of the cycle generally is associated with clinical manifestations of fever, malaise, and oral ulcerations. More rare symptoms are arthralgia, sore throat, headache, lymphadenitis, and cutaneous ulcerations. The disorder may begin in infancy, or may become evident at any age. The etiology is obscure. The oral manifestations, often described as subacute gingivitis, stomatitis, recurrent oral eruptions, or oral infections, are an outstanding feature of the cyclic neutropenia and may be the major problem of the patient[499]. In the neutropenic phase there is often a flare-up of an existing gingivitis, and other lesions may appear along the marginal gingiva. In the 10-year-old boy seen here the change consisted primarily of a fiery red, well-demarcated zone around some of the teeth as is clearly seen on the permanent first molar.

Cyclic neutropenia

Another characteristic gingival manifestation seen in patients with cyclic neutropenia is a localized punched-out lesion as seen in the illustration opposite. It is from an 8-year-old boy, who had suffered from gingivitis 1 year before admission. For 4 months the gingivitis was treated with local procedures. In some periods the patient was without symptoms, which led to a suspicion of a cyclic neutropenia. During a gingival flare-up, in the form of multiple ulcerations along the marginal gingiva, a blood examination was performed. The white blood cell count was 4,520, somewhat below the normal value, and the differential count revealed only 33 percent neutrophils, also below the normal value. As the drop in white blood cells was periodic, a diagnosis of a cyclic neutropenia was made. A number of patients with cyclic neutropenia have had the tentative diagnosis made on the basis of gingival ulcerations occurring in an asymmetric location, a feature which is typical of a systemic background. In recent years a number of children with no prior history of drug intake have been reported with marked persistent neutropenia, the so-called congenital neutropenia, associated with severe gingival inflammation, excessive tooth mobility, and extensive loss of alveolar bone[119, 378].

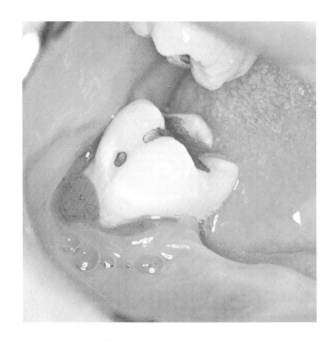

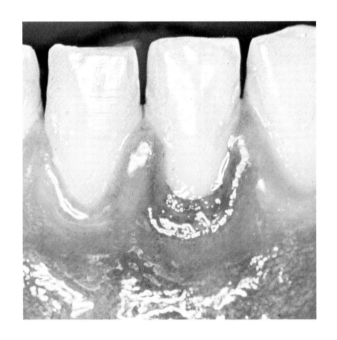

Chronic idiopathic neutropenia

Apart from cyclic neutropenia, there exists a chronic neutropenia of unknown etiology. The symptoms are recurrent febrile episodes of upper respiratory tract infections and occasional slight enlargement of the liver and spleen. The blood picture shows a marked neutropenia, but spontaneous remission may occur. Oral lesions may be present[315] as in the 9-year-old boy shown here, who was referred because of a subacute gingivitis, loosening of the permanent mandibular first molars, and recurrent aphthous ulcerations. All primary molars had been extracted due to loosening. He had an ulcer on the lower lip, an inflamed, spongy gingiva, and an unhealthy-looking oral mucosa. A blood count revealed a neutropenia with a marked lymphocytosis. The patient died 2 years later in connection with an appendectomy. Children with chronic idiopathic neutropenia will often suffer from advanced periodontitis[451]. A very rare condition is familial benign chronic neutropenia, inherited as an autosomal dominant trait, which is also associated with periodontal disease[138]. It has been suggested[34] that the severity of the periodontal lesions in patients with neutropenia may result from a depressed host defense associated with a unique virulent microbial flora.

MENTAL DISORDERS

Selfinflicted injury

Many patients practice undesirable habits which involve the oral structures. Most of these selfinflicted lesions are located to the gingiva. They are also known as gingivitis artefacta or factitial gingivitis. The following procedures have been recognized as etiologic factors for selfinflicted gingival injuries: pressure from fingernails, extended use of dummysucking, and application of pencils, pocket knives etc. to the gingiva[68]. It is characteristic of the selfinflicted lesions that (1) they are found in young people, (2) they are mostly of a bizarre configuration with sharp outlines on an otherwise normal background and (3) the grouping and distribution of the lesions are unusual and in positions that can easily be reached by the patient's hand[536]. The selfinflicted lesions are much more frequent among girls than among boys. They often appear against a background of personal unhappiness and depression and are an outward expression of a deeper disorder. The patient shown here is an 11-year-old boy, who was nervous and had the habit of pressing a pencil against the gingiva causing the retraction seen in the picture.

154

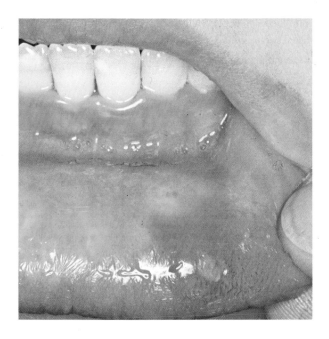

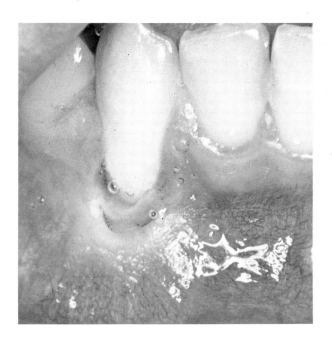

155

Amyotrophic lateral sclerosis

Amyotrophic lateral sclerosis is a chronic progressive disease of unknown etiology characterized by atrophy and fasciculation of the wasted musculature. Men are affected more frequently than women. This progressive motor disorder affects the motor cortex, nuclei of the brain stem, the pyramidal tracts, and the anterior horn cells of the spinal cord. On early examination muscular weakness with muscle atrophy and fasciculations is usually first noted symmetrical in the small muscles of the hands. At this stage of the disease hyperactivity of the deep reflexes is a striking and characteristic finding. The muscles of the palate, pharynx and tongue commonly are affected. Weakness of these muscles develops in practically all cases in the terminal stages of the disease and is the initial symptom in approximately 25 percent[368]. Speech may be slurred and eating solid food and taking liquids causes choking[471]. The tongue is atrophic, reduced in strength[151], and the constant fasciculation of the muscles gives it the appearance of a bag of worms[368]. Movements of the tongue are performed weakly and the patient may be totally unable to protrude it from the mouth. The illustration shows fasciculation in the tongue in a 60-year-old woman with amyotrophic lateral sclerosis.

Paralysis of hypoglossal nerve

The hypoglossal nerve, or the twelfth cranial nerve, is the motor nerve to the muscles of the tongue. Unilateral injuries of the nucleus in the medulla or the peripheral nerve may result in paralysis and atrophy of the muscles of one-half of the tongue. The injuries may be caused by acute anterior poliomyelitis, infectious polyneuritis, neurofibromatosis, and syringobulbia (syringomelia). The affected tongue deviates toward the paralyzed side when protruded, and movements toward the normal side are absent or weak. However, the patient is able to push the tongue against his cheek on the paralyzed side. When the tongue lies on the floor of the mouth it may deviate or curl slightly toward the healthy side, and movements of the tongue toward the back of the mouth on this side are impaired[368]. If the paralysis is not accompanied by atrophy, the tongue may appear to bulge slightly and to be higher and somewhat more voluminous on the paralyzed side, but when atrophy supervenes, the paralyzed side becomes smaller and the tongue may become curved toward the paralyzed side with a sickle-shaped deformity[35]. The illustration shows a left hypoglossal nerve paralysis in a 54-year-old woman.

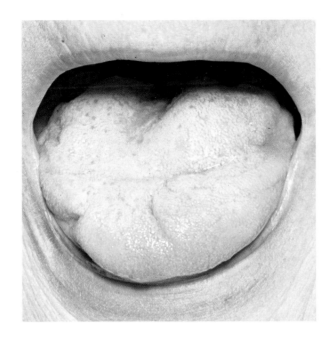

DISEASES OF THE PERIPHERAL NERVOUS SYSTEM

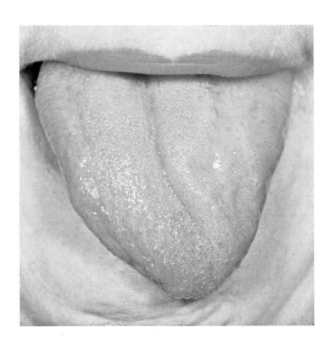

Melkersson-Rosenthal syndrome

Patients exhibiting unilateral facial paralysis, swelling of the face, and plicated tongue are grouped together under the name of Melkersson-Rosenthal syndrome (MRS). The syndrome is often seen in incomplete (oligosymptomatic) form. It affects men and women equally, and there is no racial predilection. Women are chiefly subject to the disease in the 1st, 2nd and 6th decades, whereas men predominate in the other decades[263]. Although many etiologic factors have been suggested, the etiology in most instances remains obscure. In our own department some patients have been cured of the swellings after removal of dental foci. The swelling, which is the dominant feature of the syndrome, is non-tender and non-pitting, and may assume large proportions. Miescher's cheilitis granulomatosa should be considered an oligosymptomatic form of MRS. The illustration is of a 29-year-old woman, who was referred for recurrent swellings of the lower lip and a plicated tongue. A labial biopsy revealed non-caseating, epitheloid cell granulomas. A granulomatous cheilitis may be associated with an asymptomatic Crohn's disease of the lower gastrointestinal tract[79]. In another study, 16 patients with MRS were investigated for evidence of Crohn's disease with negative results[600].

Melkersson-Rosenthal syndrome

The facial edema comprising the lips and/or the nearby regions of the face may appear abruptly from one day to the next[263]. The facial and labial edema in MRS will in most patients recur during spring and fall, finally resulting in permanent enlargement of the lips. Besides the labial and facial regions, the buccal mucosa may be involved. It becomes prominent, slightly erythematous and lobulated with shallow furrows, a "bucca lobata"[493]. These features are clearly seen in the illustration opposite which is of a 48-year-old woman. For 6 years the patient had suffered, besides the buccal changes, from a marked macrocheilia and a plicated tongue. Also the palate may be the seat of manifestations of MRS in the form of rather firm granular enlargements. The edematous swelling may extend to the soft palate, the uvula and the peritonsillar area. When the tongue is affected, the result is a macroglossia, a glossitis granulomatosa. This condition should not be confused with the third characteristic component of the syndrome: the plicated tongue, which is found in less than half of all patients with MRS[263]. The plicated tongue associated with MRS has the same clinical features as the plicated tongue found in 7 percent of the population not affected by MRS (p. 222).

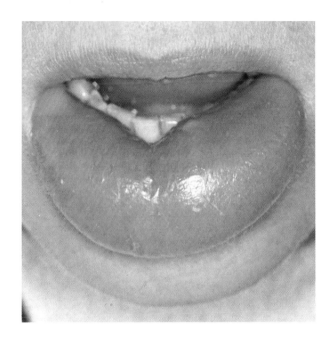

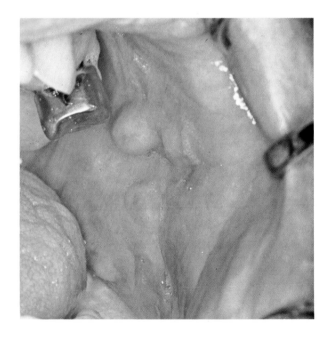

Melkersson-Rosenthal syndrome

Gingival manifestations of MRS are rarely reported, although they may be more frequent than hitherto believed. Because of their inconspicuous presentation they may often be overlooked. In a material of 30 patients with MRS (complete and abortive forms) had gingival lesions[601]. The gingival symptoms reported by the patients were recurrent swellings which gradually became more or less permanent, soreness of the "gums", and occasional gingival bleeding during toothbrushing. The gingival changes consist primarily of distinct, small, irregular, bluish-red, edematous swellings affecting the interdental papillae, the marginal and the alveolar gingiva. In some patients the swellings are less demarcated because of a marked diffuse, edematous enlargement as is obvious in the illustration opposite. The patient is a 36-year-old woman who was referred for an atypical gingivitis. It was striking that the gingival manifestations mainly appeared in the anterior part of the mouth. The histologic examination revealed non-caseating epithelial cell granulomas, associated with aggregations of lymphocytes, changes which are regarded as the prototype of histologic findings in MRS[263].

DISEASES OF THE CIRCULATORY SYSTEM

Malignant granuloma

"Malignant granuloma", "lethal midline granuloma", or "midline malignant reticulosis" is a destructive, usually fatal lesion of unknown etiology. The malignant granuloma is seen mainly among younger and middle-aged people; approximately two-thirds of the patients are men. The prodromal stage is characterized by infection in the upper respiratory tract and nasal obstruction with a purulent discharge. The destructive process has its primary site in the nasal cavity, the palate[91], or in the retromolar area. Some cases have presented following the extraction of a tooth. From these areas the adjacent structures are destroyed by direct extension of the necrotic process. In the later stages a mutilating destruction makes the facial appearance monstrous by disclosing the inner structures of nose and jaws. The patient seen here is a 45-year-old woman who, for the past 6 years, has had a rhinitis and lately developed a saddle nose. Serologic tests for syphilis were negative. At the time of admission the patient had a perforation of both superior palpebrae and an extensive destruction of the soft palate.

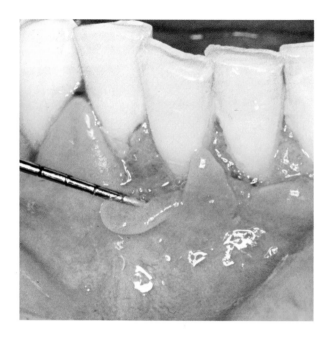

DISEASES OF ARTERIES, ARTERIOLES AND CAPILLARIES

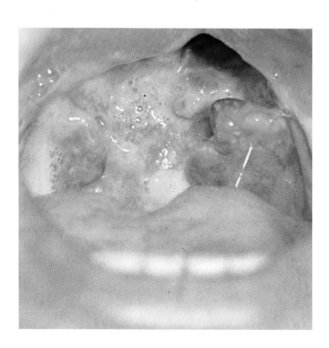

Wegener's granulomatosis

Wegener's granulomatosis is a distinct clinico-pathologic entity characterized by granulomatous vasculitis of the upper and lower respiratory tract, together with glomerulonephritis. Although the cause is unknown, the disease is generally considered a hypersensitivity disorder because of the granulomata, inflammation of vessels, and glomerulonephritis, as well as circulating and apparently deposited immune complex seen in some patients[183]. Wegener's granulomatosis is a distinct entity within the group of systemic vasculitis syndromes. It is a rapidly fatal disease characterized by a necrotizing granulomatosis of the respiratory tract, showing marked arteritis associated with granulomatous lesions of the kidneys and lungs. Wegener's granulomatosis begins with a chronic nasal or pulmonary infection, or oral changes. These consist of either ulcerations or granulomatous lesions of the gingiva[272]. In the patient shown opposite, a 58-year-old woman, the disease began with a painful palatal ulceration and crust formation in the nose. Treatment with corticosteroids improved the condition and the palatal ulceration healed. After 11 years lung infiltrates were demonstrated and the treatment was supplemented with cytostatics. The condition, however, deteriorated and the patient expired.

Hereditary hemorrhagic telangiectasia

Hereditary hemorrhagic telangiectasia, also known as Osler's disease and Osler-Rendu-Weber syndrome, is a disorder of the capillaries and smaller blood vessels characterized by telangiectatic lesions, hereditary occurrence, and hemorrhagic diathesis[214]. The vessels are without elastic tissue and are easily engorged causing repeated hemorrhage from the abnormally dilated vessels. The disease is not caused by formation of new vessels but is due merely to dilatation of existing vessels. Hereditary hemorrhagic telangiectasia is not extremely rare except among Negroes. The disease is transmitted as an autosomal dominant trait affecting both sexes equally. Cutaneous, visceral, and mucosal structures are involved, and three different types of telangiectases are found: (1) pin-point; (2) spider-like; (3) nodular. The lesions are bright red, violaceous, or purple. When a glass slab is pressed upon them, they blanch. Often the patients are pale and may have a history of fatigue and weakness caused by bleeding from the gastrointestinal tract with resultant anemia. Telangiectases are observed most frequently on the facial skin, especially on the cheeks and nasal orifices, as seen in the patient pictured here, a 30-year-old woman. Telangiectasia of the nasal mucosa may give rise to recurrent epistaxis.

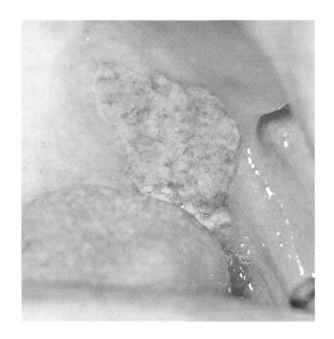

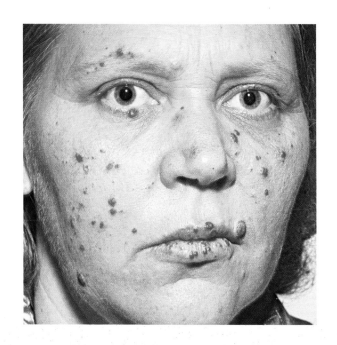

Hereditary hemorrhagic telangiectasia

Oral manifestations frequently are observed in hereditary hemorrhagic telangiectasia, and recognition of oral lesions often has led to the correct diagnosis. Bleeding from the mouth is second in frequency to epistaxis. The oral telangiectases rarely are seen before puberty and increase in size and number with advancing age[299]. The mucocutaneous junction of the lips and the tongue are most frequently involved. On the tongue, the tip and anterior dorsum are the favored sites, as seen in the illustration which is from the patient seen above. The palate, gingiva, and buccal mucosa may be similarly, though less frequently affected. Hemorrhage from the gingiva and buccal mucosa occurs less frequently than from the lips and tongue. A fatal outcome has been reported after gingival bleeding. If the gingiva is the site of telangiectases, toothbrushing should be carried out with great care. It is interesting that tooth extraction does not necessarily lead to undue bleeding[366]. From a differential diagnostic point of view, angiokeratoma corporis diffusum and lingual varicosities should be considered. However, in the former the lesions are smaller, and in the latter the lesions are confined to the ventral surface of the tongue (p. 164).

Sublingual varicosities

The undersurface of the tongue in 68 percent of individuals past the age of 60 years shows hemispherical, small, round, purplish-colored elevations, which often appear in the form of chains over ectatic venous vessels[170]. The condition has been called "lingual phlebectasias", "sublingual varices", or "lingual varicosities"; occasionally the term "caviar tongue" is used. The varicose veins occur lateral to the sublingual veins extending toward the margin of the tongue, as seen in the illustration, which is from a 66-year-old woman. When located in the floor of mouth the varicosities are found near the ostia of the sublingual glands. A statistically significant relationship between cardiopulmonary disease and sublingual varicosities has been found in persons 30 to 59 years of age[170]. In spite of the fact that varicosities of the legs and the tongue increase with age, a highly significant relationship between the two diseases was found when age was held constant. Lingual varicosities may be part of the disease of multiple phlebectasia which affects the jejunum and scrotum[447]. It has been postulated that the lingual varicosities are due mainly to diminished tissue support secondary to degeneration of the elastic fibers.

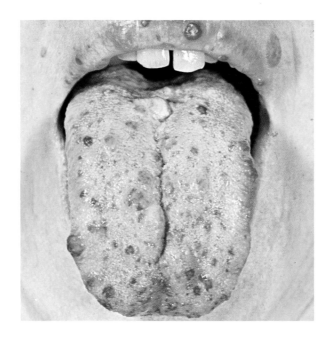

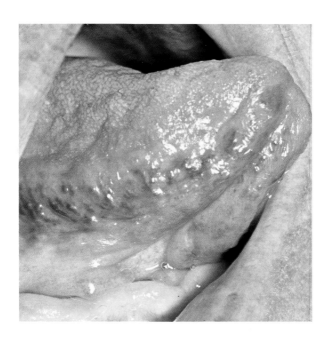

Influenza

Influenza is caused by a virus which enters the organism through the respiratory tract. After an incubation period of 1 to 2 days, the following symptoms appear: fever, headache, aching muscles and joints, nausea, and prostration. Usually, influenza is a benign condition, but when it occurs in a pandemic, such as the Spanish Disease in 1918–1919, the prognosis becomes serious. In the ordinary type of influenza, oral manifestations are extremely rare. It is known, however, that pain was a prominent oral symptom and oral ulcerations were observed during the 1918–19 pandemic[89]. From the pandemic of Asian influenza in 1957–58 there is a detailed report from Finland[589] on the oral manifestations. The most frequently observed changes were enanthema and hyperemia of the soft palate. A number of cases had an easily bleeding hypertrophic gingivitis involving the entire gingiva. Furthermore, herpes-like ulcerations and glossitis were observed in some cases. The most severe change consisted in an overall stomatitis associated with large fibrincovered erosions. Such a case is illustrated here in a 20-year-old Dane, who suffered from Asian influenza in 1958.

DISEASES OF THE DIGESTIVE SYSTEM

Toothbrushing-induced gingival ulcerations

Gingival ulcerations may occur in association with acute necrotizing gingivitis or as a manifestation of a systemic disease such as neutropenia (p. 150), benign mucous membrane pemphigoid (p. 240) or lichen planus. Selfinflicted injuries are most often located to the gingiva (p. 154). In 1979, attention was called to some unusual gingival ulcerations found in a Danish material of 38 patients with an average age of 23.4 years; most patients were teenagers[486]. It is characteristic that the lesions are diagnosed among well-motivated individuals with excellent oral hygiene. The toothbrushing is carried out with great force with horizontal movements leading to loss of epithelium, in a half-moon shape, of the marginal gingiva. In more advanced lesions, as in the 19-year-old man shown here, there is a substantial loss of gingival tissue and even of bone. It is a characteristic finding that the top of the interdental papillae is unaffected, which may be explained by the horizontal movements, whereby the papillae, protected in the interdental space, are not hurt. The disease has also been called traumatic ulcerative gingival lesion[29]. An important differential diagnosis is acute necrotizing gingivitis[69].

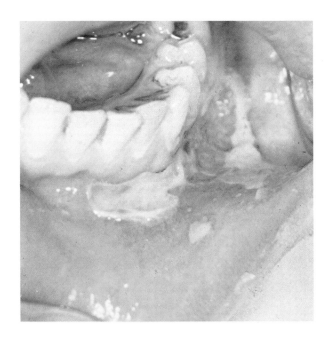

GINGIVAL AND PERIODONTAL DISEASES

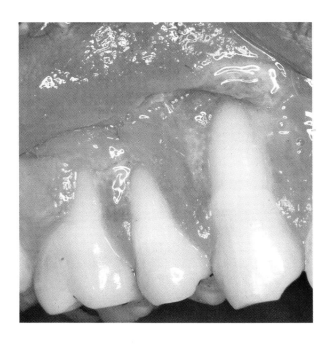

167

Idiopathic gingival fibromatosis

The syndrome of idiopathic gingival fibromatosis and hypertrichosis has been known for more than a century. It has been described under several names, such as "congenital macrogingivae", "elephantiasis gingivae", "hereditary gingival fibromatosis", and "idiopathic gingival hyperplasia". The syndrome is inherited as an autosomal dominant trait with good penetrance[214]. There is no sex predilection. Patients suffering from the syndrome sometimes may have difficulty closing their lips because of the marked gingival enlargement. Occasionally, there is a general coarseness of features resembling the facial changes seen in acromegaly. The gingiva usually enlarges in infancy, or even as late as the 9th year. The vestibular and lingual aspects of the teeth frequently are completely covered by thick, firm to soft, pink or red, resilient gingiva. In children, the affected areas have a smooth or finely stippled surface, but later they may acquire papillary projections[474]. Usually, the gingival enlargement is greater in the maxilla than in the mandible. The patient seen here is a 26-year-old woman who had had the enlarged gingiva for many years. The second molar and the two premolars were almost buried in the gingiva and had nearly total loss of alveolar bone.

Idiopathic gingival fibromatosis

The patient described above returned to the hospital 4 years after the first visit, presenting the changes illustrated. Each interdental papilla was enormously enlarged and none of the incisor teeth had any bony support. A clinical examination of the body revealed a moderate hypertrichosis. The degree of hypertrichosis in patients with idiopathic gingival fibromatosis is extremely variable. Although intelligence is normal in most patients with the syndrome, mental retardation has been recorded by several authors. Gingival fibromatosis may also be associated with multiple hyaline fibromas, or corneal dystrophy, or ear, nose bone, and nail defects and hepatosplenomegaly or microphthalmia, mental retardation, athetosis, and hypopigmentation[214]. Failure or delay in the eruption of teeth is frequent and may occur in one or both dentitions[474]. So-called partial cases have been described in which the fibromatosis develops around a particular group of teeth. Not uncommon is the symmetric fibroma of the palate which appears to be a partial type of idiopathic gingival fibromatosis. This enlargement usually originates from the palatal gingiva of the maxillary first molars, extending and increasing in width posteriorly.

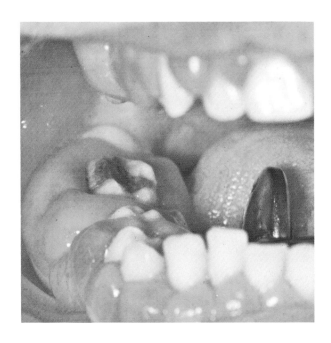

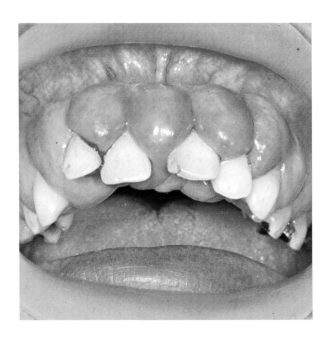

Gingival cyst

The WHO classification of jaw cysts defines a gingival cyst as a cyst arising from epithelial cell material left in the gingiva[424]. That the gingival cysts are not as rare as hitherto thought is reflected by an increasing number of case reports on the cyst. A distinction should be made between the lateral periodontal cyst, which arises within the periodontal membrane, and the gingival cyst which originates within the gingiva. Gingival cysts are most commonly found in the region between the lateral incisor and the first premolar in the buccal aspects of the jaws[365], most often in the mandible. The majority occurs in older patients. Most gingival cysts will remain as histologic phenomena. When a gingival cyst attains a sufficient size, it becomes clinically recognizable as in the illustration opposite which is from a 71-year-old woman. The cyst was surgically removed and studied histologically. The cyst lining consisted of a two- or three-layer, non-keratinized squamous epithelium. Usually the cysts are found on the attached gingiva having a dome-shaped appearance. Often there is history of a swelling which disappears when finger pressure is applied, only to reappear within a few days. The cyst lining may be squamous epithelium with or without keratinization, or a respiratory epithelium[384].

Peripheral giant cell granuloma

Most commonly known as "giant cell epulis" is a tumor-like condition usually developing from the margin of the gingiva. The term "peripheral giant cell granuloma" is to be preferred to "peripheral giant cell reparative granuloma". In a material of 173 patients with peripheral giant cell granulomas[557] it was found that the highest occurrence rate was during the period of mixed dentition. Whilst in childhood the granuloma was commoner in boys than girls, after the age of 16 the number of women affected was twice that of men. The mandible is affected somewhat more often than the maxilla, and more often in the premolar-molar region than the incisor-canine region[557]. Clinically, the giant cell granuloma is a well-defined, rather soft swelling with a purple, often slightly bluish color as in the 58-year-old man shown opposite. In most cases the lesion is found in relation to teeth, but it may be observed also on the mucosa of the edentulous alveolar ridge. Often a local irritation is demonstrable, indicating that this factor may play an important role. The tendency for recurrence is marked.

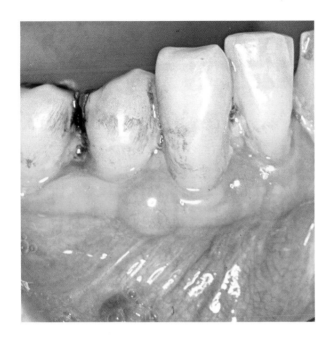

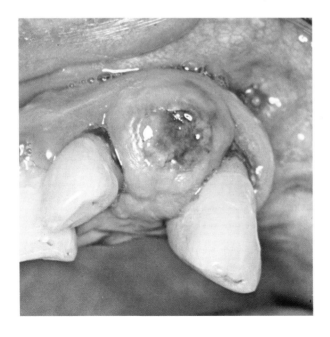

Atrophy of maxillary alveolar ridge

Denture-induced changes of the oral mucosa comprise (besides denture stomatitis, p. 62) the so-called flabby ridges and folds and redundancies in sulci. A flabby ridge or alveolar fibrosis, in German "Schlotterkamm", originates when parts of the alveolar ridge become resorbed due to excessive occlusal trauma on the denture in the affected area. It is seen more often in women than in men[291]. The area most often affected is the anterior part of the maxilla[546] but the mandible also may exhibit the fibrosis. The facial morphology may be altered as a result of the alveolar bone loss[551]. The mucosa covering the alveolar ridge becomes the site of an inflammation when the ridge is exposed to excessive trauma. The inflammation contributes further to the resorption of the alveolar ridge, which gradually is replaced by a collagenous, inflamed tissue. A flabby ridge usually is more red in color than the adjacent, normal mucosa and may sometimes be associated with a denture irritation hyperplasia, as in the case illustrated here, of a 78-year-old woman who has been wearing an upper denture for many years. Usually the flabby ridge has a rather firm consistency, depending on the degree of inflammation in the connective tissue.

Denture irritation hyperplasia

The folds and redundancies of the oral mucosa in sulci are called by different names, such as epulis fissuratum, granuloma fissuratum, and denture hyperplasia. The use of the term "epulis" should be discarded as a misnomer. As the hyperplasia is caused by irritation from a denture, the term "denture irritation hyperplasia" seems appropriate. The hyperplasia usually is seen in patients who have worn ill-fitting dentures over a rather long period of time and is more frequent in women than in men[60, 398] with the maxilla and mandible equally affected. The irritation may come from overextended flanges or from sharp margins of the denture. Most often the pressure from these ill-fitting dentures first causes a traumatic ulceration. When the ulceration heals under constant irritation, hyperplasia of the oral mucosa is most likely to occur. The majority of denture irritation hyperplasias are located on the alveolar ridge, the rest are found in the vestibular sulcus except for a few percent which are located on the lingual sulcus[398]. The hyperplasia may consist of a single flap, or there may be multiple folds and impressions from the denture as in the 65-year-old man shown here.

172

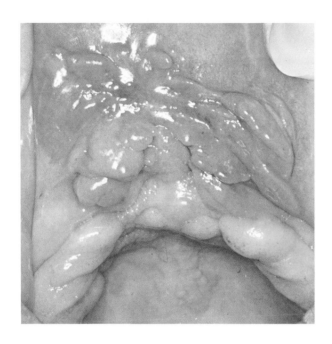

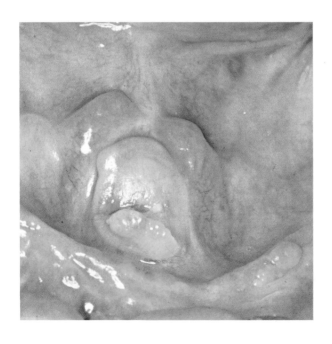

Eruption cyst

In the WHO classification of odontogenic cysts[424], an eruption cyst is defined as a cyst that lies superficial to the crown of an erupting tooth and that is lined with non-keratinizing, stratified squamous epithelium. The paucity of reports on eruption cysts is not an indication of this lesion being rare, as has been shown in a comprehensive study of 4,480 episodes of primary tooth eruption[504]. The study showed that an eruption cyst occurred in 11 percent of the infants during the eruption of the incisors and in 30 percent of the infants during eruption of the canines and molars. The eruption cyst occurs usually in childhood most often in connection with primary teeth and it is more frequent in girls than in boys. It is a blue, bluish, or blue-black translucent, elevated, compressible, dome-shaped lesion of the alveolar ridge, overlying the erupting tooth[504]. The cyst may be firm on palpation, although a fluctuation is most often found. The illustration is of an 8-year-old boy where the eruption cyst is covering an unerupted first premolar. There are some differences of opinion as to the origin of the eruption cyst. Most likely the pathogenesis is the same as for the dentigerous cyst.

Mucocele of labial salivary glands

A mucocele is the condition which arises through dilatation of a cavity with accumulated mucous secretion. The mucocele, originating mostly in relation to the minor salivary glands in the oral cavity, is a rather frequent condition, and is also known as a "mucous retention cyst". For many years it was an accepted theory that oral mucoceles were due to accumulation of mucous in the salivary glands in which the excretory duct had been obstructed. Now it is recognized that two types exist: (1) the more common mucous extravasation cyst in which mucous has extravasated into the tissues and may or may not be enclosed by granulation tissue[118]; (2) the more rarely found mucous retention cyst, in which the cavity is lined with epithelium. The first type is caused by trauma to an excretory duct or to the glandular parenchyma, leading to a rupture through which mucous seeps out into the adjacent tissue; the second is due to an obstruction of the excretory duct. Mucoceles occur most commonly in the lower lip, which tends to be exposed more often to trauma. They are soft, painless, fluctuant, well-defined swellings with a characteristic bluish appearance, as in the 8-year-old girl shown here.

174

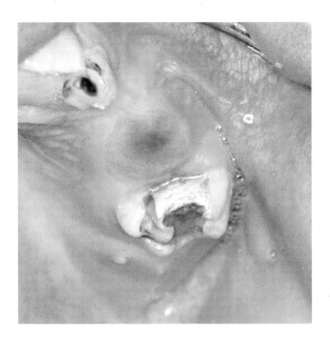

DISEASES OF THE SALIVARY GLANDS

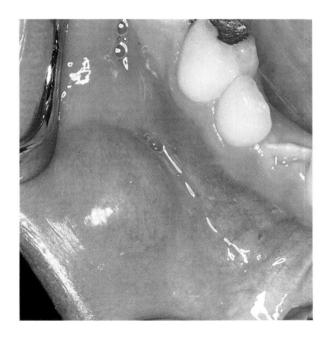

Mucocele (ranula) of sublingual gland

Ranula is the term for a mucocele localized in the floor of the mouth. It has been used because the sublingual mucoceles seem to resemble a frog's belly (ranula is diminutive of *rana*, a frog), but it is a poor term since other conditions in the floor of the mouth may have a similar appearance. Most authors today agree that ranula is nothing more than a descriptive term, relating to a cystic swelling of a translucent blue dislocation in the floor of the mouth. The term should therefore be discarded. A mucocele in the floor of the mouth usually is seen on one side. These mucoceles may stem from minor salivary glands, in which case they are small and more superficially located[118], or they may have originated from one of the sublingual glands and are then larger and more deeply situated, as in the 17-year-old girl seen here. Most sublingual mucoceles are of the mucous extravasation cyst type (see above). There is a deep-seated type, the plunging ranula. This condition has a high recurrence rate. From a number of documented cases it appears that an average of three operations, frequently involving extensive neck dissection type procedures, have been necessary before the condition was finally cured[8]. A sublingual mucocele may also be congenital[454].

Necrotizing sialometaplasia

Necrotizing sialometaplasia is a non-neoplastic, inflammatory, self-healing lesion of human salivary glands first described in the minor salivary glands of the palate in 1973[3]. Out of 33 documented cases up till 1979, 88 percent were located to the palate[343]. The average age in the same material was 46 years with a male:female ratio of 2.7:1. Clinically, the palatal lesion is characterized by a rapid growing ulcerated swelling, 1 to 2 cm in greatest dimension. In a few patients there has been bilateral affection. Histologically, the outstanding features are lobular necrosis of the salivary glands, squamous metaplasia of acini and ducts, pseudoepitheliomatous hyperplasia and prominent granulation tissue and inflammation. The picture opposite illustrates an example of a necrotizing sialometaplasia in the palate of an 18-year-old woman[422]. A week before admission the patient noticed a small, slightly painful swelling in the palate. A biopsy showed the lesion to be a necrotizing sialometaplasia and the patient was kept under observation. After 8 weeks the lesion had completely disappeared. In the past, a necrotizing sialometaplasia has, clinically and/or histologically, been mistaken as a mucoepidermoid tumor or a carcinoma. Most investigators believe the lesion is an infarctive phenomenon[343].

176

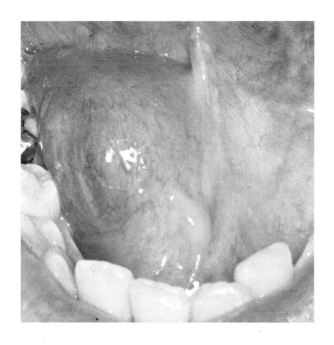

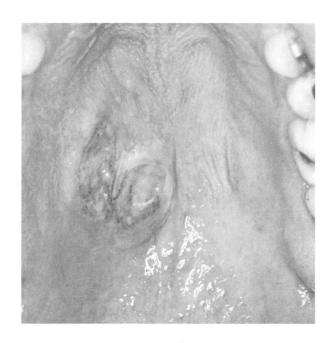

Cancrum oris

Under the names "noma" and "gangrenous stomatitis", and "infectious oral necrosis", cancrum oris has been known for hundreds of years in various parts of the world. Today the disease is mostly confined to some of the developing areas in Africa, Asia, and South America. Cancrum oris begins as an ulceration of the oral mucous membrane extending out from within and causing a well-demarcated necrosis of the overlying skin, as seen in the 8-year-old boy from South India shown opposite. Usually there is profuse salivation and an extremely foul smell. The gangrenous area separates rapidly, whereafter sequestration of the underlying bone and teeth occurs. Because of the toxic effects of the infecting organisms, the patients become seriously ill[527]. Most investigations have found a maximum incidence of cancrum oris in the 2- to 5-year-old age group; and adults are rarely affected. The disease is slightly more common in girls. *Borrelia vincenti* and *Bacillus fusiformis* are always present in the lesions of cancrum oris. In Nigeria it has been found[163] that cancrum oris is always an extension of an acute necrotizing gingivitis into the adjacent soft tissue. Diseases, such as measles, smallpox, malaria and acute herpetic gingivostomatitis, may be associated factors.

Cancrum oris

Cancrum oris usually is seen as a complication of one of the exanthematous eruptive fevers; in West Africa it is especially associated with measles. In 250 cases of cancrum oris from Nigeria measles was the predisposing acute illness in 70 percent of the cases[167, 552]. Malnutrition is also a predisposing factor, although cancrum oris is comparatively rare in frank kwashiorkor (p. 130). In two recent patients from Micronesia[225] malnutrition and sepsis appeared to be initiating factors. Although poor oral hygiene may favor the development of acute necrotizing gingivitis, the forerunner of cancrum oris, the latter may develop in children with quite good oral hygiene, and in children with no obvious predisposing illness. At one time the disease was almost fatal, but the use of sulfonamide drugs and antibiotics has reduced the mortality to about 10 percent. The improved treatment has, however, led to a considerable number of disfigured faces, presenting a challenge to the plastic surgeon. The 18-year-old Indian woman shown opposite suffered from cancrum oris as a child. The lips are destroyed, the skin blends directly with the attached gingiva, and the teeth are very irregularly placed. Also the chin shows the effect of the necrotizing process.

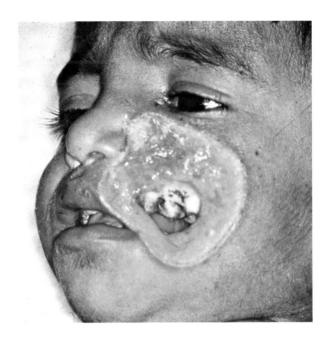

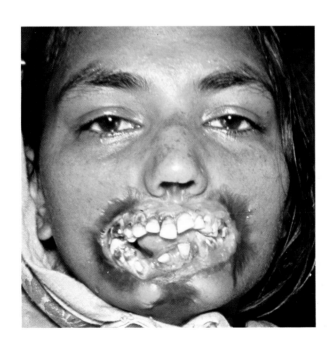

Gangrenous ulceration

Outside the tropical countries cancrum oris is extremely rare. In other countries the only destructive lesion of significance is the acute necrotizing stomatitis (p. 54). In rare cases, however, the oral mucosa may become the site of an extensive necrotizing or gangrenous lesion if the general resistance of a patient is extremely low and the oral hygiene very poor. It is well known that diabetics are more prone to develop gangrenous lesions in various parts of the body than are normal persons. The picture illustrates an alarming condition which was observed in a 66-year-old woman who, for 7 years prior to this oral examination, had suffered from diabetes mellitus and hypertension. Three weeks before admission to the hospital she noticed a swelling of the right cheek, which was followed by an ulceration. At admission the condition consisted, as illustrated, of an extensive, deep, gangrenous ulceration covered with fibrin and debris. By means of intensive local treatment and systemic use of antibiotics, a perforation to the skin was prevented, and complete healing was obtained. The development of the lesions was probably conditioned by the diabetes and by the fact that the patient was in a poor nutritional state.

Recurrent aphthous ulcerations

Known under names such as "canker sore", "aphthous ulcerations", "recurrent stomatitis", and 'recurrent aphthous ulcerations" (RAU) a condition exists which is characterized by recurrent ulcers of the oral mucosa and oropharynx. The condition varies in prevalence from 10 to 65 percent in various population samples. Women are affected more commonly that men. A definite etiologic factor has not been identified for RAU, but heredity, trauma, psychic stress, menstrual cyclus, pregnancy and history of atopic disease[595] may be associated with RAU. Humoral and cell-mediated immunity against oral streptococcal antigens and human oral mucosa appears to be features of RAU[142]. Other studies[573] have provided suggestive evidence that immune complex deposition may play some role. An early lesion of RAU is usually felt by the patient as a burning sensation. Later, when an ulcer is established, the pain may become very intense. The first attack is most commonly experienced between the ages of 10 and 20 years. After that, recurrence may take place at intervals of several years, or the patient may have many attacks each year. The patient seen here is a 32-year-old man who had had aphthous ulcers for 5 years in the location shown in the picture.

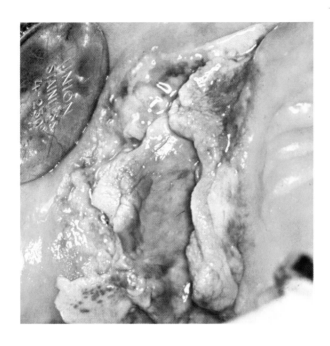

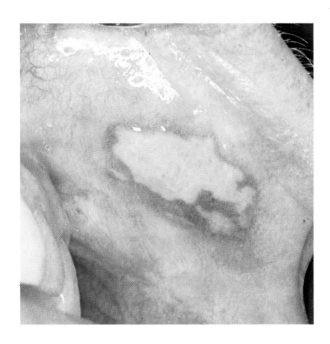

Recurrent aphthous ulcerations

In recent years there has been a discussion in the literature about the possible etiologic role of deficiencies of iron and B_{12} and coeliac diseases. Also recently some studies have clearly indicated that certain food components (figs, cheese, tomatos etc.) participate in the etiology of some cases of RAU[242, 595]. The aphthous ulcerations are seen most frequently on the labial and buccal mucosa. Next follow the tongue and floor of mouth. It is very rare to see RAU located to areas of the oral mucosa which normally are keratinized, i.e. the hard palate and gingiva. Therefore, it is understandable that the keratin-producing habit of smoking is negatively correlated with the prevalence of RAU[27]. In this connection it should be mentioned that smokers have much less RAU than non-smokers. This may be due to the hyperkeratosis of the oral mucosa induced by smoking. The RAU, which vary considerably in diameter, are well-demarcated fibrin-covered ulcerations of varying depth, surrounded by a red halo. The characteristic morphology is seen in the two illustrations opposite from a 16-year-old woman who had had recurrent lesions for 4 years. The number of ulcers usually varies from a single lesion to 5–10 ulcers. The ulcers will most often heal within 1 to 3 weeks without scar formation.

Herpetiform ulcerations

Recurrent focal ulcerations of the oral mucosa comprise (1) recurrent aphthous ulcers, (2) periadenitis necrotica recurrens, and (3) herpetiform ulcerations, the latter type having been described[122] in 1960. In a sample from London of 100 patients with recurrent oral ulcerations (ROU), 81 percent had recurrent aphthous ulcers, 8 percent periadenitis mucosa necrotica recurrens, and 8 percent herpetiform ulcerations[323]. The herpetiform ulcerations begin as small pinhead-sized erosions that gradually enlarge and eventually coalesce. The lesions may be 10 to 100 in number, involving any part of the oral mucosa. The ulcers have a diameter of 1 to 2 mm. In these features they differ from recurrent aphthous ulcers, but resemble herpetic lesions. However, the differ from herpes simplex in that the vesicular stage rarely is seen clinically, and multinucleated giant cells and a rising antibody titer against herpes simplex virus have not been recorded. The peak incidence of herpetiform ulcerations is from 20 to 29 years which is somewhat later than for recurrent aphthous ulcers. The lesions are more painful to the patients than would be expected by their size[81]. The etiology of herpetiform ulcerations is unknown. Most likely the disease is a variant of the RAU.

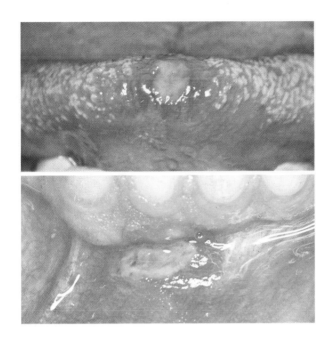

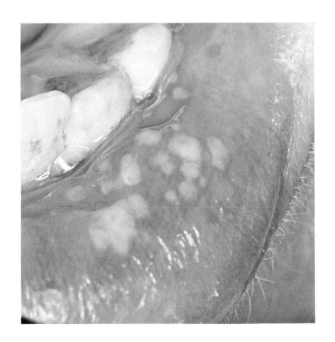

Periadenitis mucosa necrotica recurrens

Whereas recurrent aphthous ulcers will heal without scar formation, there is a condition, clinically similar to aphthous ulcers, which is characterized by a marked tendency to form scars. This condition, usually called periadenitis mucosa necrotica recurrens, has also been termed "stomatitis aphthosa recurrens cicatricicans", "Sutton's aphthae", and "neurotic ulcers of the mouth". The condition is extremely painful: so much so that several patients have attempted suicide. It seems to be more frequent in women than in men. The lesions, which most often are multiple, will begin as tender submucous nodules. Over a period of a few days the nodules enlarge, the overlying mucosa becomes necrotic, and an ulcer forms. In contrast to the recurrent aphthous ulcers, which are usually rather superficial, the ulcers in periadenitis mucosa necrotica recurrens are deep, crateriform, and may be accompanied by considerable induration, as in the 45-year-old man seen here. This patient has had unbearable pain almost constantly for 1 year and his buccal oral mucosa is marked by the scars so typical of this condition. Superimposed upon the scars is a fibrin-covered ulceration. The illustration also shows ulcerations on the inferior surface of the tongue.

Periadenitis mucosa necrotica recurrens

Some authors consider the term periadenitis mucosa necrotica recurrens to be a misnomer and believe that the lesions should be called major aphthous ulcerations because they are conveived as an exaggerated form of typical recurrent aphthae. The lesions in periadenitis mucosa necrotica recurrens last longer, are larger in size, and recur more frequently. Like recurrent aphthous ulcerations, the lesions in periadenitis mucosa necrotica recurrens are rarely found on the gingiva. The tongue is rather frequently affected, although the extenive lesion on the inferior surface of the tongue shown above is somewhat unusual. The patient opposite was a 73-year-old man who had had ulcerations of most areas of his oral mucosa for 2 years. The etiology of the disease is obscure. Significant hemagglutinating antibodies to oral mucosa have been found in 80 percent of patients with periadenitis mucosa necrotica recurrens, in 72 percent of patients with RAU, but only in 10 percent in controls[326]. IgG and IgM have been demonstrated in the cytoplasm of epithelial cells in biopsies of ulcers from patients with RAU, periadenitis mucosa necrotica recurrens and Behçet's syndrome indicating a relationship between the three entities[325].

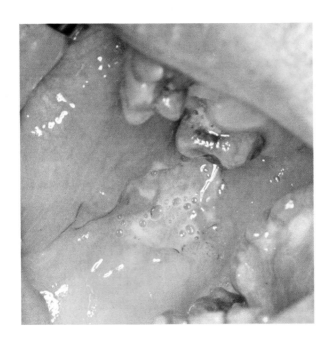

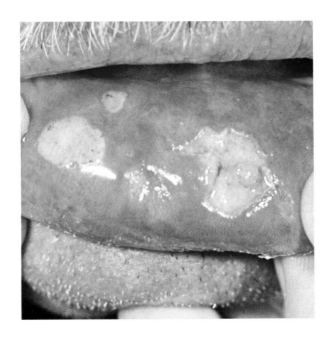

Gingival cysts in newborns

Small cysts or nodules on the oral mucosa are very common in newborns and infants. They often are referred to as Epstein's pearls or Bohn's nodules. There are two favored sites for the lesions, i.e. the palate and the mucosa covering the alveolar ridge. Clinical studies of 1-day-old full-term infants have demonstrated that 80 percent have cysts of the palatal or alveolar mucosa, or both[98]. The most common location is along the median palatine raphe (65 percent), followed by the maxillary alveolar mucosa (37 percent) and the mandibular alveolar mucosa (20 percent). The cysts are found less frequently in Negro newborn infants than in Caucasian newborns[287]. The cysts on the alveolar mucosa, usually called gingival cysts, vary in size from 1 to 3 mm. They are white, slightly elevated, and often multiple, as in the 4-month-old girl shown here. Histologically, the cysts contain concentric layers of keratin. They arise from islands of odontogenic epithelium and undergo a transition to squamous epithelium with subsequent epidermoid cyst formation. Treatment of the cysts is not indicated, since they disappear spontaneously within a few months by opening to the surface mucosa.

Dermoid cyst of floor of mouth

A dermoid cyst is a developmental cyst consisting of a fibrous wall lined with stratified epithelium and containing dermal appendices such as hair follicles, sweat glands, sebaceous glands, and teeth. Dermoid cysts also may be found in the oral cavity, although they are quite rare. When the cyst is located above the mylohoid muscle, the tongue may be displaced superiorly causing difficulties in eating as in the 17-year-old boy shown opposite. The cyst fluctuated and its natural color made it quite easy to distinguish from a ranula (p. 176). The histologic examination showed a keratinized cyst lining and the presence of sebaceous glands. When the cyst is located below the mylohyoid muscle, the soft tissue is distended in the submental region and, in cases of larger dermoids, there is a bulging in the floor of the mouth. Although a developmental anomaly, the dermoid cyst in the floor of mouth is rarely seen at birth and usually appears in adults before the age of 35[338]. There is no sex predilection. The cysts are painless, slowly growing lesions that vary in size from a few millimeters to 10 cm.

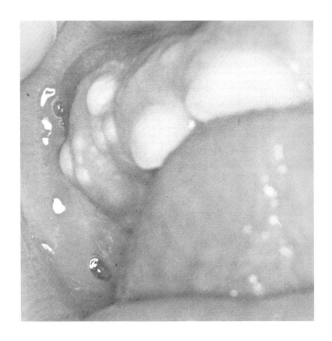

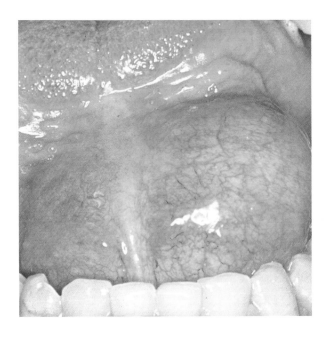

Sublingual lymphoepithelial cyst

The lymphoepithelial cyst is a soft tissue epithelial cyst associated with lymphoid tissue. The paucity in the literature of reported cases of the lymphoepithelial cyst is probably due to the small size and asymptomatic nature of the lesion. The lymphoepithelial cyst has been called a branchial cyst, a branchiogenic cyst, or a pseudocyst. It is assumed that the lympho-epithelial cyst develops by proliferation of epithelium which has been isolated within lymph nodes during development. The majority of the lymphoepithelial cysts are located to the floor of the mouth as in the 11-year-old boy opposite. Next in frequency is the tongue[111]. The cysts, which are covered by a normal appearing mucosa, are freely movable. Usually the color of the cyst is yellow or yellow-white. The lesion, which usually is found between 20 and 50 years of age, is asymptomatic. The lymphoepithelial cyst is small, rarely exceeding 1.5 cm. Histologically, the cyst is lined with a stratified squamous epithelium, which usually is parakeratotic. Surrounding the cyst lining are masses of lymphocytes often arranged in a follicular pattern. Some investigators[304] consider the lymphoepithelial cyst as an oral tonsil comparable to the hypertrophic foliate papilla (p. 218).

Exfoliative cheilitis

Exfoliative cheilitis has been defined as a chronic superficial inflammatory disorder of the vermillion border of the lips characterized by persistent scaling[472]. The majority of the patients are teen-aged girls or young women[80], many of whom show evident emotional disturbance or atopy. No sensitivity to sunlight or to chemical agents appear to be involved. The illustration shows a typical example of the lesion. It is of a 22-year-old man who had been complaining of periodic attacks of scaling, peeling and cracking of the lower lip together with a lesser degree of involvement of the upper lip[566, 568]. There had been a preceding period of dryness of the lips. Both lips appear slightly swollen with masked vertical folds. The lower vermilion border is covered by a brown scaly layer with some crusting in the vertical folds. The upper lip is similarly affected in limited areas. The patient was observed for some months and a cyclic nature of the lesion was established. For some weeks the lips would be normal and then, often associated with anxiety and pressure of work, desquamating scales would appear. The patient could himself strip off the discolored scaly tissue and the cycle would begin again (By courtesy of Dr. W. R. TYLDESLEV, Liverpool, and Peter Wolfe, Publisher).

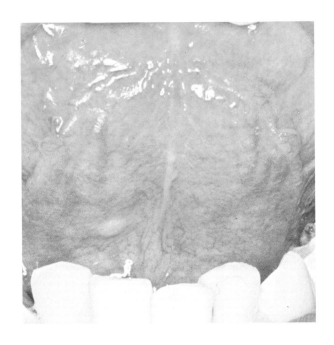

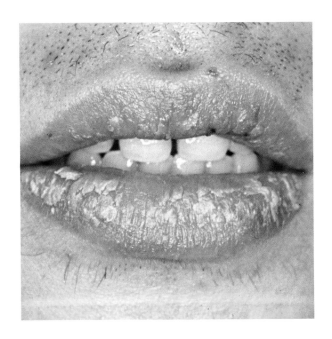

Leukoplakia of buccal mucosa

Leukoplakia is a whitish patch or plaque that cannot be characterized clinically or pathologically as any other disease and it is not associated with any physical or chemical causative agent except the use of tobacco[28, 592]. The prevalence of leukoplakia varies in different parts of the world depending upon prevailing habits[416]. In Sweden, the prevalence of leukoplakias, except for those caused by snuff, is 3.6 percent[24]. Leukoplakias are seen more often in men than in women, and usually are restricted to older age groups[582]. The leukoplakias are divided into homogeneous and non-homogeneous comprising erythroleukoplakia, nodular leukoplakia and verrucous leukoplakia[28]. Erythroleukoplakia and the nodular type of leukoplakia, which in most instances are associated with a candidal infection, are also referred to as speckled leukoplakia or speckled erythroplakia. Most leukoplakias are of the homogeneous type, although wrinkling, like cracked mud, or a delicate pattern of fine cristae occasionally may be observed. Such cristae, due to the use of tobacco[428], are seen in the illustration, which is of the buccal mucosa of a 60-year-old man who was a heavy cigarsmoker. Tobacco-induced leukoplakias are often reversible. Spontaneous regression of leukoplakias has been reported.

Candida-infected leukoplakia of labial commissure

Under the heading of chronic hyperplastic candidiasis (p. 58) a condition is discussed which is characterized by whitish areas associated with red (atrophic) and yellow (ulcerated) areas. The patient seen opposite is an example of a *Candida*-infected lesion, where the white component dominates. The picture is of a 49-year-old man who, for 3 years, had an itching sensation in the left commissure. By close scrutiny of the picture very small white nodules can be identified, some of which are in areas of atrophic mucosa. These nodules may enlarge whereby the lesion becomes a nodular (speckled) leukoplakia (p. 196). Leukoplakias are, more often than hitherto throught, the seat of a *Candida*-infection. In an English material of 53 patients with candidal leukoplakia[21], tobacco smoking and denture wearing appeared to be important local factors in the etiology of candidal leukoplakias. In a Danish study[282], 48 patients with so-called "speckled" leukoplakia were subjected to antifungal treatment after the diagnosis of a *Candida*-infection had been established. The treatment in all cases changed the speckled type to the common type with a homogeneous, whitish, slightly wrinkled surface.

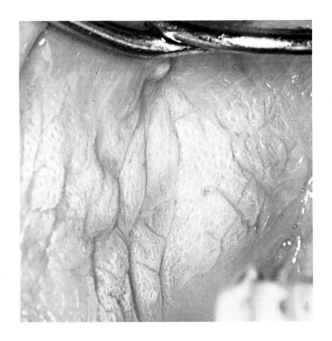

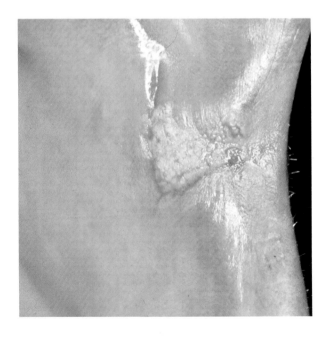

Leukoplakia of labial mucosa

The habit of placing snuff in the labial or buccal sulcus is common in several countries: Sweden, Denmark, South Africa, Sudan, and the U.S.A. In a Swedish epidemiologic survey, snuff-induced leukoplakia occurred with a prevalence of 8 percent[24]. A 55-year-old Dane with a snuff-induced leukoplakia is shown opposite. He kept snuff in the mandibular labial groove 8 hours a day for 30 years. The leukoplakia, which presents the same type of fine cristae as in the lesion illustrated on p. 190 is stained brown by the snuff. Whereas snuff-dipping in the U.S.A. not too rarely may lead to development of oral cancer, especially among women[596], the snuff-induced leukoplakias observed in Denmark and Sweden only rarely exhibit premalignant changes. In countries where tobacco is chewed, oral leukoplakia also may develop where the tobacco quid is kept. In some parts of North India the quid, composed of betel and tobacco, is kept in the mandibular labial sulcus[367]. A recent study in U.S.A. has shown that among 1119 high school students 10 percent used smokeless tobacco. Fifty-two percent of the users had whitish lesions (leukoplakias) of the labial mucosa[223]. In England an increased prevalence of leukoplakias has been found among coal miners who chew tobacco in comparison with those who only smoke[565].

Leukoplakia of labial mucosa

The illustration opposite shows clearly the difference in the mode of reaction of the vermilion border and the labial mucosa to leukoplakiogenic agents. The picture is of a 69-year-old man who smokes eight cheroots daily. On the labial mucosa there is a homogenous leukoplakia, whereas the vermilion border is the seat of a crusty lesion. The majority of leuko-plakias on the labial mucosa are well-defined and of a homogenous uni-form type; most of them are found on the lower labial mucosa. In a considerable number of patients with leukoplakias of the labial mucosa the lesions have a pattern of very fine, delicate, keratinized striae. An interesting observation has been made in a neuropsychiatric hospital[58], where 11 percent of 750 patients had the so-called cigarette smoker's lip lesion. Of the patients displaying this type of leukoplakia on the labial mucosa, 62 percent had lesions on both upper and lower labial mucosa. The authors state that the lesions are caused by smoking the cigarette nearly to the end. The patients are able to do this consistently because their pain threshold has been heightened by tranquillizers, which partially accounts for the insensitivity to the pain caused by such smoking.

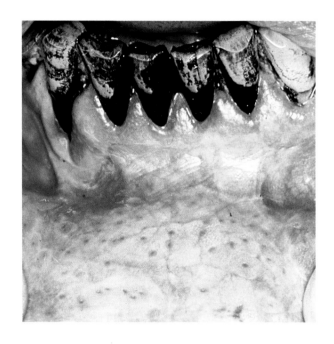

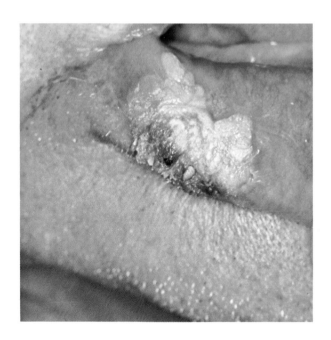

Leukoplakia of tongue

After their most frequent location, the buccal mucosa and commissures, the leukoplakias are found, in a Danish sample, in descending order, on the alveolar ridge, tongue, buccal grooves, floor of the mouth, labial mucosa, inferior surface of tongue, hard palate, and margin of the tongue[470]. In the buccal mucosa and commissures the lesions often occur bilaterally and symmetrically. Leukoplakias affecting the tongue may be located at the margin, the dorsum or the inferior surface. In larger materials of leukoplakias, those of the tongue account for about 5–8 percent. When the leukoplakia is located on the dorsum of the tongue, the papillae disappear. A serologic examination should always be carried out in cases of lingual leukoplakias, because it has been reported that late syphilis predisposes to the development of leukoplakia in this location. The 47-year-old woman seen here had, however, a negative Wassermann reaction, and she had never smoked. The leukoplakia should then be classified as idiopathic, as it was not possible to demonstrate any etiologic factors. Leukoplakias of the tongue may occur either as a diffuse involvement of the dorsum or as a well-demarcated homogenous patch as in the present case. It is important in the differential diagnosis to exclude early development of lichen planus.

Leukoplakia of floor of mouth and sublingual surface

In a material of 368 Danish patients with oral leukoplakias, 13 percent had leukoplakias located on the floor of the mouth and/or the ventral surface of the tongue[430]. Almost half of the lesions had a corrugated appearance, like a beach at ebbing tide, as in the illustration opposite which is from a 60-year-old woman who smokes 10 cheroots daily. The sex distribution is interesting for the floor of the mouth leukoplakias because women account for 71 percent of the leukoplakias in the floor of the mouth, whereas they account for only 37 percent in other locations[430]. With regard to tobacco habits the analysis revealed that the floor of the mouth group had a statistically significant higher percentage of cheroot-smokers than did the groups representing other locations. Leukoplakias affecting the floor of the mouth and the ventral surface of the tongue in patients in southern England caused discomfort of some kind in 51 percent[306], whereas the Danish material showed a remarkable paucity of symptoms. Also in contrast to the Danish findings is the higher risk of malignant transformation found in the English material. It is interesting to note and difficult to understand why floor of the mouth leukoplakias are extremely rare in India where smoking habits are so prevalent[367].

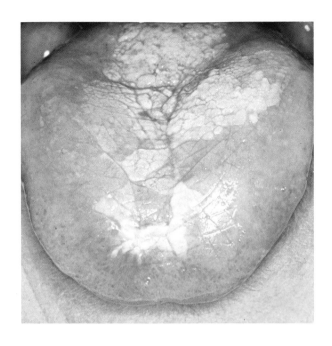

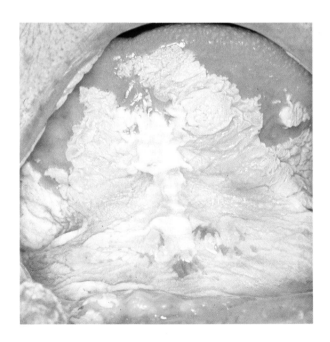

Nodular (speckled) leukoplakia of labial commissure

A number of oral leukoplakias present a picture of white patches on an erythematous background giving a nodular or "speckled" appearance recently called erythroleukoplakia[519a]. It has been shown that the nodular leukoplakias in two-thirds of the cases are associated with epithelial dysplasia or carcinoma[429]. Care should be taken not to mistake for nodular leukoplakias the traumatized leukoplakias which are quite frequent in the commissural area. The 63-year-old man seen here, a heavy smoker, has nodular (speckled) lesions in both right and left commissures, both revealing epithelial dysplasia. As mentioned (p. 58), a nodular leukoplakia may have a superimposed *Candida*-infection, which is the case with this patient. The malignant transformation of oral leukoplakia is probably not as frequent as was thought previously. Several follow-up studies of oral leukoplakias carried out in recent years have found a frequency of malignant transformation ranging from 1 to 6 percent[416]. However, a recent American study[519a] has found a malignant transformation rate of 18 percent. It is often difficult to compare directly the various follow-up materials as these materials are derived from different sources, mostly selected samples, and variable approaches have been applied to the treatment.

Erythroplakia of buccal mucosa

Erythroplakia is used analogously to leukoplakia to designate lesions of the oral mucosa that present as bright red patches or plaques that cannot be characterized clinically or pathologically as any other condition[28]. Occasionally, whith plaques are observed in or adjacent to the lesion or in other parts of the oral mucosa[511]. The histopathologic features of erythroplakia are marked epithelial atrophy associated with epithelial dysplasia, carcinoma in situ or squamous cell carcinoma[509]. Erythroplakia, a rare lesion most often seen on the penis, may occur on the buccal mucosa (most frequent oral site) and the soft palate, occasionally extending down the glosspalatine fold, and, very rarely, on the tongue. In a study of 67 asymptomatic floor of the mouth cancers and carcinoma in situ, it was found[354] that an erythroplakic component occurred in 97 percent. The patient seen here is a 55-year-old woman who had a typical erythroplakia located mainly on the left buccal mucosa and extending on to the alveolar ridge. A biopsy from the red area in the left cheek revealed a mild epithelial dysplasia. During a long follow-up period the lesion first faded almost completely away, but ultimately a carcinoma developed 13 years after the patient was examined the first time.

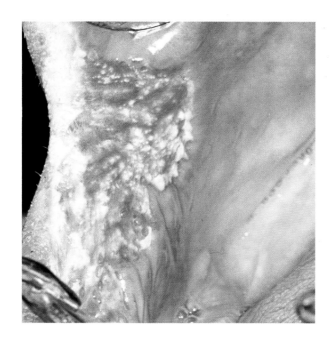

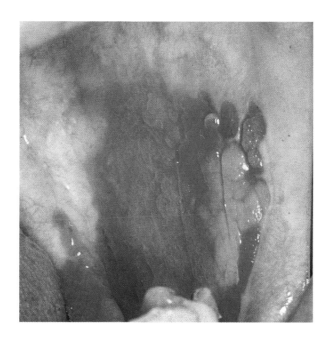

Leukoedema of buccal mucosa

Leukoedema is a chronic condition in which the oral mucosa has a gray, opaque appearance. On the smooth surface a grayish film seems to hang like a veil. It can be scraped off, but will soon reappear. Leukoedema has been considered a variant of normal mucosa in which there is incomplete shedding of parakeratotic cells. Prevalences of leukoedema have been established in several epidemiologic surveys and range from 0.02 percent in India[367] to 16.9 percent in New Guinea, where a strong relationship has been demonstrated[417] between leukoedema and smoking of sticks (imported tobacco wrapped in newspaper). In a Swedish epidemiologic study[26], leukoedema was found in 49 percent. Leukoedema was significantly more prevalent among individuals with some daily tobacco habit than among those without. The wide variation in prevalence rates must be ascribed to differences in criteria. The illustration which is of the right buccal mucosa of a 30-year-old Papuan man, shows a grayish-bluish-white, coarsely wrinkled surface. The patient smoked many tobacco sticks daily. Histologically, leukoedema is characterized by an increase in thickness of the epithelium, which is the site of a marked intracellular edema. The flattening and swelling of the outer cells can be a form of abortive keratinization with abnormal forms of keratohyalin granules[610a].

Smoker's palate

"Smoker's palate", "nicotinic stomatitis", and "leukokeratosis of the palate" are synonyms for the condition described here as smoker's palate as nicotine has nothing to do with the hyperkeratosis characterizing the lesion. An epidemiologic study of 20,333 unselected Swedes[24] showed a prevalence of 1 percent. In India the highest prevalence has been 0.3 percent[367] except for areas with reverse smoking where the prevalence of palatal keratosis is 9.5 percent[426]. Smoker's palate is observed most frequently in pipe smokers. Probably both chemical and thermic factors are of significance. In the early stages, the condition is characterized by a reddening of the palate which soon assumes a diffuse, grayish-white, occasionally wrinkled appearance. Later the mucosa becomes thickened and the site of nodules with a small red dot in the center representing the opening of the duct outlets. A typical example is illustrated in the palate of a 57-year-old man who had smoked many pipes daily for 30 years. Cessation of smoking will cause improvement of the condition. The western type of palatal leukokeratosis is not precancerous. The palatal changes found in reverse smokers differ from the ordinary smoker's palate clinically as well as histologically.

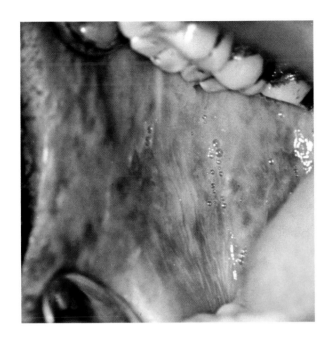

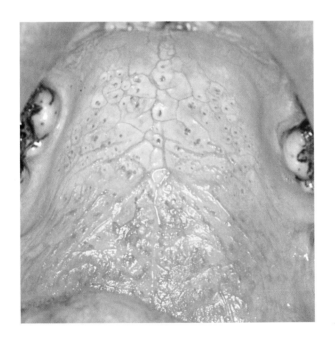

Focal epithelial hyperplasia

The term focal epithelial hyperplasia was introduced[19] in 1965 to signify certain multiple, nodular elevations of the oral mucosa observed among American Indians in New Mexico, USA and in Brazil. Since then the disease has been found not infrequently among Indians in many Latin American countries and among Canadian and Greenland Eskimos[440]. The highest prevalence so far (35.8 percent), has been found among Eskimos in Angmagssalik, Greenland. Isolated cases have now been reported from many countries in Europe and Africa[477]. So far, no case have been reported from Asia, apart from Asia minor. The lesions in focal epithelial hyperplasia are slightly elevated, flat, sessile, and soft. Usually the surface in finely stippled or slightly keratotic; most often the color is like that of the adjoining mucosa. When the mucosa is stretched, some lesions tend to disappear. Their size is usually between 0.1 and 0.5 cm. Most commonly seen in the lower labial mucosa, they sometimes extend out on the vermilion border; the next most frequent sites are the buccal mucosa, commissures, and labial mucosa of the upper lip. In Eskimos, however, more than 50 percent are located to the tongue, as in the 35-year-old Eskimo from Angmagssalik shown here (Courtesy of Dr. F. PRÆTORIUS, Copenhagen, Denmark).

Focal epithelial hyperplasia

The picture illustrates a typical case of focal epithelial hyperplasia in the buccal and labial mucosa in an 11-year-old Danish Caucasian girl. She also had similar lesions on the right side and on the border of the tongue. There have been many suggestions concerning the etiology of focal epithelial hyperplasia, ranging from local irritating factors to vitamin deficiencies. Evidence of a viral infection has been found based on microscopic[117], electron microscopic, and immunofluorescence examinations[441]. Immunohistochemical studies have demonstrated the presence of papilloma virus antigen in focal epithelial hyperplasia[439]. The virus has been found to be human papillomavirus Type 13 (HPV 14)[414]. Focal epithelial hyperplasia has been known before 1965, but was described under names such a papilloma, verruca, or multiple polypus hyperplasia. The concept of focal epithelial hyperplasia as a conditions seen nearly exclusively in children and young adults is not supported by the findings in the Eskimo population in Nanortalik, where the highest prevalences were found in the age groups above 30 years. Spontaneous regression or disappearance of the lesions has been observed by several investigators.

200

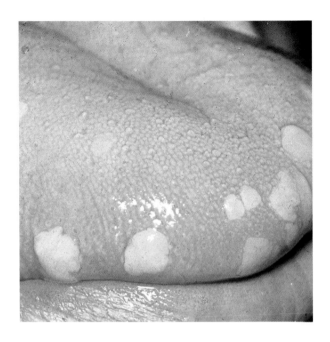

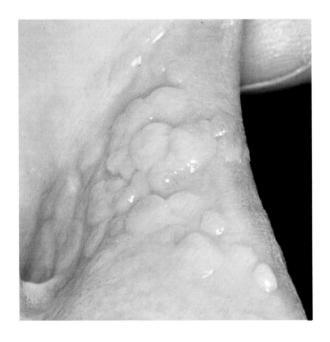

201

Geographic stomatitis

Whereas the concept of geographic tongue is old, dating back to 1831, the idea of a similar lesion occurring in other parts of the oral mucosa was not suggested till 1955 when such a condition was called "erythema migrans affecting the oral mucosa". Other terms for the same condition are "exfoliatio areata linguae et mucosae oris"[312] and "geographic stomatitis"[267]. As the other parts of the oral mucosa may be affected without tongue involvement it seems preferable to use the term geographic stomatitis. A representative example is shown in the illustration opposite. It is from a 25-year-old woman in whom the lesions were incidentally discovered by her dentist. As can be seen in the picture the lesions are characterized by a half-moon shape of an elevated white line which borders up to a red area. A biopsy of one of the lesions showed the white line to consist of a hyperplastic epithelium with parakeratosis with migration of inflammatory cells. There were no indications of a *Candida*-infection. After a spontaneous disappearance the lesions recurred within a few months affecting this time the attached gingiva of the mandibular incisors. There have never been lesions on the tongue. The etiology of geographic stomatitis is unknown.

Denture stomatitis with multiple intramucosal fistulae

Denture stomatitis with multiple intramucosal fistulae of the palate seems to form an entity with characteristic clinical and histologic features. It was first described in 1979 on the basis of findings in 13 denture-wearing patients, all women[480]. The patients show small, yellowish areas in the hard palate, which sometimes resemble sebaceous glands. When erythema is present in adjacent areas, the yellow spots are difficult to identify. On pressure with a blunt instrument a whitish creamy material can be expelled through multiple openings in the palatal mucosa. The palatal lesions are located posterior to the palatal rugae and anterior to the junction between the hard and soft palate and anterior to the posterior edge of the denture as well. The main part of the lesions are located towards the middle of each half of the palate. When guttapercha points are inserted into the openings they appear through another opening, which demonstrates that different openings are connected with each other as is clearly seen in the illustration of a 63-year-old woman. Also an erythema is present. The origin of the intramucosal fistulae may be explained by proliferations and invaginations of the surface epithelium caused by the pressure from a long-standing denture wearing.

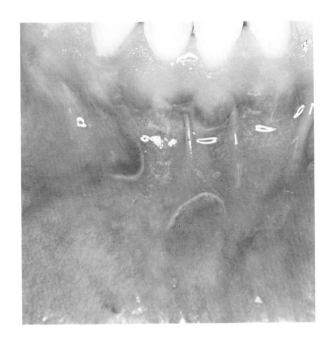

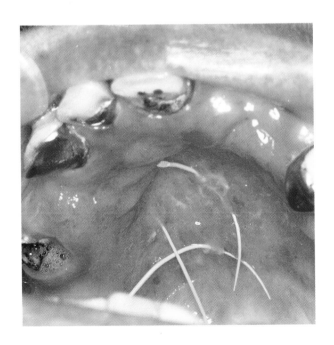

Glassblower's white patch

Glassblowers are known to present with oral manifestations in the form of white lesions on the buccal mucosa, and thickening, dark discolorations, leukoplakic and verrucous changes of the labial mucosa. Changes of the dental hard tissues include discoloration, fracture, and abrasion. The white patches have earlier been referred to as leukoplakias[289]. As the use of the term leukoplakia has been suggested to comprise only idiopathic white lesions and tobacco-associated lesions[28], the changes seen in the oral mucosa of glassblowers should not be called leukoplakias. Oral changes related to the occupation of glassblowing have been examined in 74 Danish glassblowers, consisting of 44 active glassblowers and 30 past glassblowers. In addition, 15 non-glassblowers were examined. All three groups worked in the same department of mouth-blown glassware in Holmegaards Glassworks. White patches of the oral mucosa occurred in 23 percent of active glassblowers, but did not occur among past or non-glassblowers[484]. An example of such a glassblower's white patch in a 45-year-old man is seen opposite. He went on vacation and when he returned 3 weeks later the white patch had completely disappeared. Histologically, the white lesions revealed morsicatio buccarum-like changes. It appears likely that the white patches develop mainly as a result of mechanical traumas.

Oral submucous fibrosis of buccal mucosa

Submucous fibrosis may be defined as an insidious, chronic disease affecting any part of the oral cavity and sometimes the pharynx as well. Although occasionally preceded by and/or associated with vesicle formation, it is always associated with a juxtaepithelial inflammatory reaction followed by a fibroelastic change of the lamina propria, with epithelial atrophy leading to stiffness of the oral mucosa and causing trismus and inability to eat[431]. The condition has been reported mainly among East Indians, but the author has diagnosed submucous fibrosis in Sri Lanka, Malaysia, Nepal, Singapore, Thailand, South Vietnam, and among Indians living in Africa and in the Fiji Islands. Epidemiologic studies have shown a prevalence between 0.2 and 1.2 percent in India and 0.5 percent among Indians in South Africa. The most common initial symptom is a burning sensation in the mouth, often experienced when the patient is eating spicy food. Other frequent early symptoms are blisters, ulcerations, or recurrent stomatitis. At examination some patients may present vesicles, especially in the palate, but the striking feature is the blanching of the mucosa, as seen in the 50-year-old Indian man shown here. The affected area also has a superimposed leukoplakia.

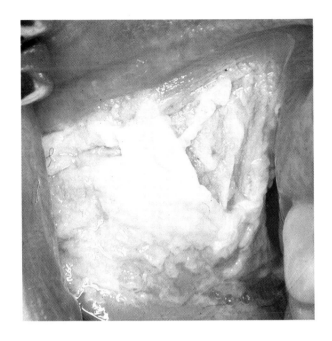

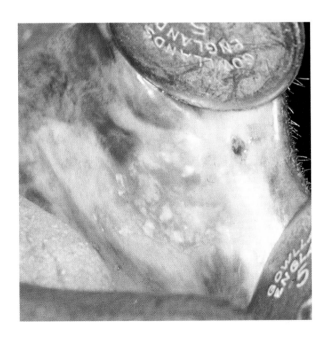

Oral submucous fibrosis of palate

The blanching in this condition is due to a loss of the pigmentation present in the oral mucosa in most Indians. The whitening often takes place in spots, so that the mucosa acquires a marbled appearance. Quite often leukoplakic patches appear and, occasionally, fiery red erythroplakic areas are seen. After varying periods of time the patients complain of stiffening of certain areas of the oral mucosa, leading to difficulties in opening the mouth and in swallowing. Clinically, palpation reveals the presence of fibrous bands, especially in the palate, faucial pillars, buccal mucosa, and lips. The oral mucosa usually is involved symmetrically. The fibrous bands in the buccal mucosa run in a vertical direction, whereas in the soft palate the fibrous bands radiate from the pterygomandibular raphe or the anterior faucial pillar and have a scarlike appearance as in the 45-year-old Indian woman seen here, who had an advanced degree of submucous fibrosis. The uvula is markedly involved in the later stages; it shrinks, appears as a small fibrous bud also seen in the illustration and the entire isthmus faucium is reduced. The cause of submucous fibrosis is obscure. However, the habit of betelnut chewing has been found to be highly correlated with the occurrence of submucous fibrosis[227, 514].

Oral submucous fibrosis with carcinoma

There is a certain evidence that submucous fibrosis represents an oral precancerous condition. First, epithelial dysplasia has been found in 14 percent of 220 cases of submucous fibrosis; second, the frequency of oral leukoplakia in cases of submucous fibrosis is six to eight times higher than in a control group. Third, it has been found in South India that among oral cancer patients, almost half also had submucous fibrosis, a frequency far exceeding the 1.2 percent with submucous fibrosis found among the general population in the same area. Fourth, that a follow-up study of patients with submucous fibrosis has demonstrated a higher malignant transformation rate than in individuals without the disease[427]. The following pathogenesis is conceivable: in patients with submucous fibrosis, the oral epithelium becomes atrophic and thereby probably more vulnerable to carcinogens, which in India are so often present in the form of chewed tobacco. The atrophic epithelium first becomes hyperkeratotic, a change eventually followed by epithelial dysplasia. From then on, carcinoma may develop at any time. The picture is from a 28-year-old Indian man who had developed a commissural cancer on the basis of a submucous fibrosis, which also has caused a marked atrophy of the tongue papillae.

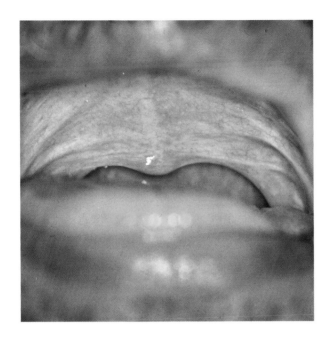

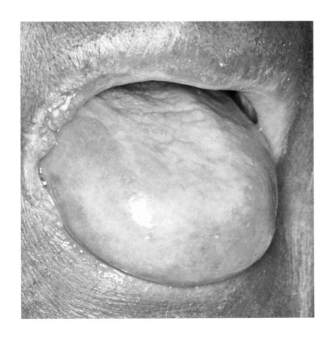

Linea alba

The linea alba appears as a more or less thick line on the buccal mucosa at the level of the occlusal plane and is pale gray or white in color. The illustration opposite shows a typical linea alba in a 48-year-old woman who was very tense. It has been suggested by one investigator that the linea alba is caused by the buccinator muscle pressing the mucosa over the cusps of the maxillary posterior teeth and into the line of occlusion[317]. Despite the frequent occurrence of the linea alba, few studies have been concerned with the lesion. In one of these studies 27 men and 7 women were selected from a group of 256 young adults examined for the presence of linea alba[292]. Linea alba was detected in 13 percent of the sample of 256. Its presence did not appear to be associated with insufficient horizontal overlap or roughness of the buccal cusps. However, the linea alba seemed to be the result of interaction of two factor: the presence of continuous negative intraoral pressure and the position of the mandible. Cytologic studies of color and morphologic differentiation indicate that some degree of keratinization of the epithelium overlying the linea alba, in part, accounts for its whitish appearance[292].

Cheek-biting

Cheek-biting may be performed unconsciously. The condition is also called "morsicatio buccarum" or "pathomimia mucosae oris". Prevalence studies have only been carried out in selected samples. In a Danish sample of 8,589 persons of all ages, 0.5 percent had either lip- or cheek-biting[505]. In a South African sample of 1,255 pupils from reform schools (for children in need of care) the prevalence was 4.6 percent[611]. The lesions vary in appearance according to etiology. The cheek-biting lesions are characterized by a distinct desquamation of the affected epithelium. They have a whitish, rough, macerated appearance and are diffusely outlined. The illustration is of a typical example from a 17-year-old girl who was very nervous and tense. Her lesions also exhibited superficial erosions. The target of cheek-biting is the linea alba, which is squeezed back and forth. Often the habit is combined with bruxism. When the lesions are caused by cheek-sucking, the clinical appearance is different. The oral mucosa exhibits whitish-grayish, lustreless patches. In more severe cases petechiae may be observed in the lesions. The selfinflicted oral lesions should be differentiated from leukoplakia and candidiasis.

208

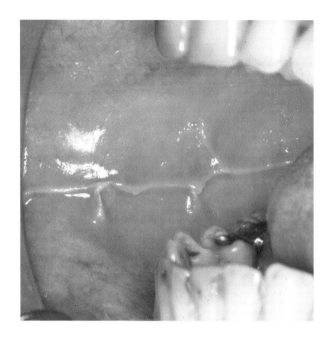

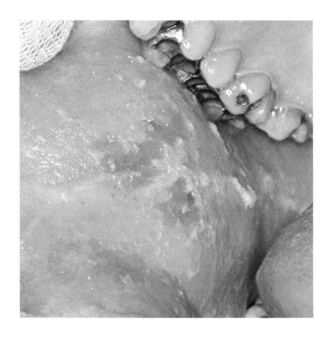

Lip-biting

It is not only the cheeks which may become the site of selfinflicted lesions caused by biting or sucking. The illustration opposite is of a typical example of the result of lip-biting in a 15-year-old girl who admitted to the habit of biting her lip. From a purely clinical point of view the lesion resembled a white spongue nevus (p. 270). In contrast to the cheek lesions shown above, the lip lesion is characterized by a fine stippling. Whereas the biting-type of lesions are characterized by an irregular flaky desquamation of the epithelial layer intermingled with minute small erosions, as seen in the picture above, the sucking-type of lesions have whitish-grayish patches of the mucosa with some degree of stippling. Also histologically there are differences between the biting and sucking type of lesions[254]. In a material of 17 patients referred by dental and medical practitioners, only one patient was referred under the correct diagnosis. The reference diagnoses varied from leukoplakia, candidiasis, and cheilitis to lesions of unknown origin. Lesions caused by lip- as well as cheek-biting may also resemble chemical burns (p. 247), leukoedema, white sponge nevus, and reaction of mucosa to dentifrices.

Pyogenic granuloma

The pyogenic granuloma of the oral cavity is most frequently located on the gingiva, for which reason it has been called an "epulis", often with the name "telangiectaticum" attached because the lesion is rich in small vessels. The pyogenic granuloma is an exaggerated response, in the form of excess granulation tissue, to minor trauma not related to any specific infectious agent[296]. The granuloma occurs almost equally in both sexes, but some authors report a slightly higher frequency in women. It occurs in all ages, but in about 60 percent of instances it involves individuals between 11 and 40 years of age[15]. A study of a large series of oral pyogenic granulomas has demonstrated that 75 percent occurred in the gingiva, with the rest located in the buccal mucosa, lip, tongue, palate, mucobuccal fold, and the frenum[62]. The pyogenic granuloma is found most often on the vestibular aspect of the anterior part of the jaw, with a preference for the maxilla. Clinically, the pyogenic granuloma is a soft, pedunculated lesion with a fiery red color and a glossy surface. Quite often the granulomas exhibit ulcerations covered with fibrin, as in the 14-year-old boy seen here. These granulomas always have a tendency to bleed copiously.

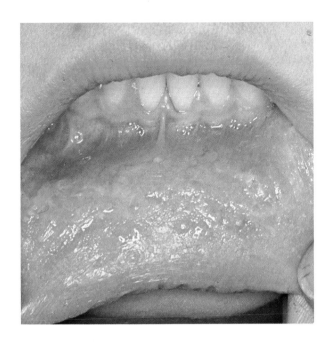

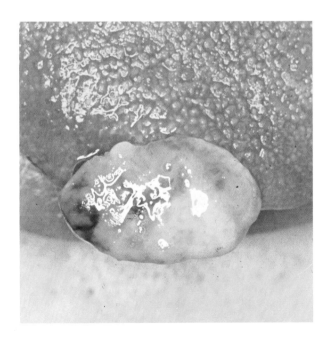

Eosinophilic granuloma of oral mucosa

Almost as rare as the eosinophilic bone granuloma is an eosinophilic granuloma located on the oral mucosa which is a distinct entity unrelated to histiocytosis X (p. 140). The lesion has also been called traumatic granuloma of tongue[608]. Of 15 cases previously reported, 13 were men most in the middle age. Fifteen have been located on the tongue, one on the palate, and one on the lip[510]. Two cases located to the gingiva have since been reported[559]. Most of these granulomas have been ulcerated. The ulceration is probably due to the moist environment and frequent traumatization[255]. The illustrated case is of a 51-year-old woman who, 4 months before admission, had several small, red spots on eyelids and hands; furthermore there had been oral ulcerations. The lesions have appeared and disappeared spontaneously in 2- to 3-week periods. At admission, the patient had an ulceration on the upper labial mucosa. A biopsy revealed changes consistent with the diagnosis of an eosinophilic granuloma with numerous eosinophils and a marked histiocytic proliferation. Following the biopsy the lesion healed rapidly. After 1 more week an ulceration appeared on the right lateral border of the tongue as seen in the illustration opposite.

Melanoplakia

Melanin pigmentation of the oral mucosa may be due to increased amounts of melanin with normal numbers of melanocytic cells or to increased numbers of melanocytic cells (nevi and melanomas)[244]. The first can be divided into group (1) lesions associated with a systemic or a local factor and (2) lesions without an identifiable etiologic factor (idiopathic). Belonging to systemic factors are melanin pigmentation caused by Addison's disease (p. 130), Albright's syndrome, Peutz-Jeghers' syndrome (p. 284), and medication with antimalaria drugs (p. 290); also belonging to the first type is racial pigmentation. Particularly, the gingival pigmentation has been the subject of several investigations. Studies of Negroes[149] and Greenland Eskimos[275] have shown pigmentation of the gingiva in 60 and 98 percent, respectively. Apparently there is no direct correlation here between the color of the skin and the gingiva. The second type comprises localized areas of increased amounts of melanin in the oral mucosa variously termed ephelis, focal melanosis, and melanoplakia. An example of such idiopathic melanin spots is given in the illustration opposite of the buccal mucosa in an 84-year-old woman with fair skin. For such changes the term oral melanotic macules has been suggested.

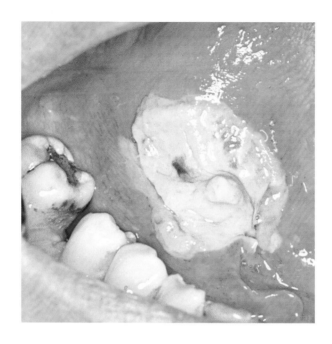

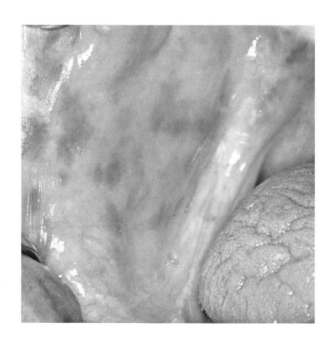

213

Smoker's melanosis

In 1977, a Swedish study revealed a strong correlation between gingival melanin pigmentation and smoking[243]. In a Swedish unselected population 10 percent had melanin pigmentation of the oral mucosa[25]. The anterior labial gingiva in the mandible was the most frequently pigmented location. The presence of melanin pigmentation was positively correlated to tobacco smoking. The smoking related oral pigmentation, smoker's melanosis, could thus be calculated at a prevalence of 19 percent among smokers and the total frequency of smoker's melanosis was calculated at 7 percent. A later investigation in Japan studied the dose-response relationship between tobacco consumption and gingival pigmentation among lead workers with no signs of metal poisoning[18]. The group of workers was examined every year for the presence of gingival melanin pigmentation over a 4-year period. At first and last examination 17 and 25 percent among those smoking more than 10 cigarettes a day had a gingival pigmentation in contrast to the non-smokers who had a prevalence of 0 and 2 percent[18]. Furthermore, it was found that the gingival pigmentation increased significantly with tobacco consumption. The picture illustrates a 64-year-old Danish man who has smoked 20 cigarettes a day for at least 30 years.

Verruciform xanthoma

Verruciform xanthoma[507] is an uncommon lesion of the oral mucosa which was first recognized[507] as an entity in 1971. Since the first description a total of 26 cases has been reported. The lesion has been diagnosed at a variety of ages. The clinical appearance varies from red through yellowish-red to gray or white with a rough, pebbly, sometimes crateriform surface. The lesion, which is always well-circumscribed, has either a sessile or a pedunculated base. The favored location of the lesion is the lower alveolar ridge either on the crest of on the buccal or lingual aspects[507]. It appears to be slow growing. Also the gingiva has been the seat of verruciform xanthoma in several cases[377]. Histologically, the verruciform xanthoma is covered by a stratified hyperparakeratotic squamous epithelium of a papillary appearance with deep crypts. The connective tissue papillae are dominated by foam cells containing lipid granules. It has been suggested[617] that epithelial degeneration precedes and ultimately causes the formation of foam cells. The illustration opposite shows a verruciform xanthoma on the hard palate in a 48-year-old man. At admission the lesion was red. A smear showed *Candida* hyphae and antimycotic treatment was given, resulting in a whitening of the lesion.

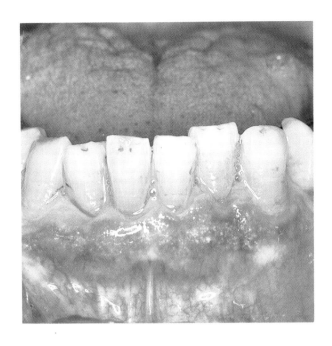

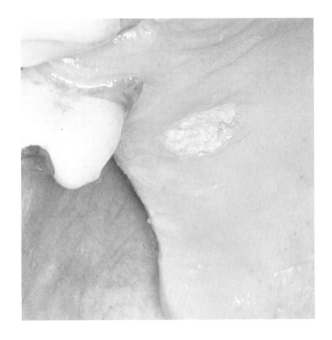

Geographic tongue

This condition, also described under the names of "exfoliatio areata linguae", "glossitis exfoliativa marginata", "glossitis migrans", and "benign migratory glossitis", occurred with a prevalence of 9 percent in an unselected Swedish population of 20,333[24]. In a sample of 70 patients with the disease, 13 percent had a familial background[39]. Among 6090 Iraqi schoolchildren (6–12 years) geographic tongue was found in 4.3 percent[206]. In geographic tongue the surface of the tongue becomes the seat of multiple zones of desquamation of the filiform papillae in several irregularly shaped but well-demarcated areas. The desquamated areas are red with slighly elevated margins, white, or yellowish. The fungiform papillae are conspicuous because of the loss of the filiform papillae. Over a period of days and weeks, the bald spots and the whitish margins seem to migrate across the surface of the tongue by healing on one border and extending on another. The picture illustrates an early stage of a geographic tongue in an 18-year-old woman. The white, elevated margins are due to heavy accumulation of inflammatory cells in the upper part of the epithelium. Forty percent of the patients with geographic tongue will also have a plicated tongue[494].

Geographic tongue

The patient shown opposite, a 67-year-old woman, shows a more advanced stage of a geographic tongue where the tongue papillae have been shed in a well-demarcated area. An extensive investigation in Israel[443] has demonstrated a simultaneous occurrence of geographic tongue, seborrheic dermatitis, and spasmodic bronchitis in children below the age of 2 years. A prolonged study revealed that a considerable number of these children developed a plicated tongue. The etiology of geographic tongue is unknown; a number of factors have been proposed, but none has been established. An Australian study suggests that geographic tongue is a sign common to those patients who have a tendency to develop recurrent acute inflammatory disease on surfaces in contact with the external environment (for example, asthma or rhinitis), whether they are atopic or not[351]. A photographic series has demonstrated a tendency for students with geographic tongue to have more severe lesions when under emotional stress than when comparatively calm. Among psychiatric patients it was found that the prevalence of geographic tongue was approximately six times higher among the mentally ill than among the students[453].

216

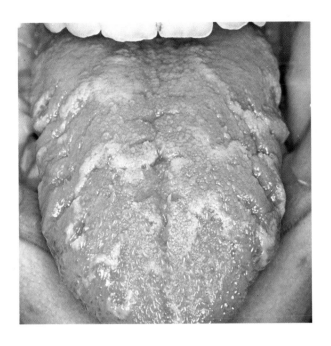

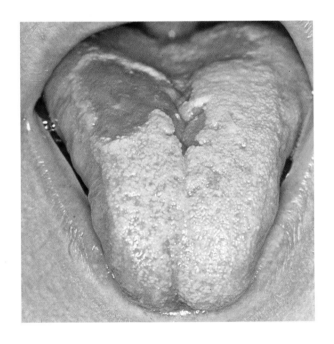

Median rhomboid glossitis

For many years it has been an acceptable assumption that median rhomboid glossitis, a well-demarcated, deep red area devoid of tongue papillae, is a developmental anomaly due to a failure of withdrawal of the tuberculum impar during the development of the tongue. The illustration from a 38-year-old woman is a characteristic example of what previously was thought to be a median rhomboid glossitis. Several investigators have now suggested that the median rhomboid glossitis is the result of a localized chronic *Candida*-infection[604]. Local factors as tobacco smoking and denture wearing apparently favors the local proliferation of *Candida albicans* on the dorsum of the tongue[20]. Some investigators have introduced the concept of a localized atrophy of tongue papillae in front of the terminal sulcus[24] and some have suggested the term "central papillary atrophy of the tongue" (CPA)[182], but have not succeeded in distinguishing clearly between this atrophy and the localized candidiasis. The CPA has been found to be relatively common in diabetic patients[178], and is also seen in denture wearers, but is no more in those wearing dentures than in non-denture wearers. The prevalence rate of CPA is found to be 1.3 percent in a South African population[182] and 1.4 percent in a Swedish population[24].

Hypertrophy of foliate papilla

The foliate papillae, located posteriorly on the lateral surface of the tongue, just anterior to the palatoglossal muscle, may occasionally become irritated, not uncommonly leading the patient to the dentist in a state of cancerophobia. The size of the foliate papillae varies considerably. In some individuals they are barely noticeable ridges, whereas in others they consist of marked rounded projections[521]. Symptoms from the foliate papillae may be due partly to an upper respiratory infection and partly to irritation. The complaints arise usually in women in the second half of life. The patients are often edentulous, and the mandibular dentures may have traumatized the area of the foliate papillae, which then starts swelling. The patient shown is a 43-year-old man who has pronounced swelling of one foliate papilla. As the core of the foliate papillae consists of lymphoid tissue, it is easy to understand that they may enlarge when other parts of the lymphoid apparatus in the pharynx react. The enlargement of the papillae renders them susceptible to mechanical irritation. The conditions has also[304] been called "foliate papillitis" or "tonsilla linguae lateralis" or "oral tonsils".

218

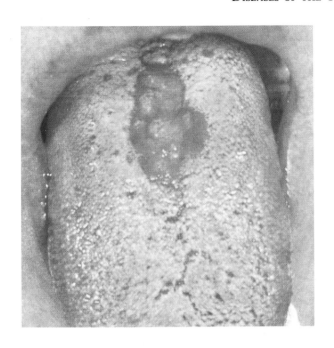

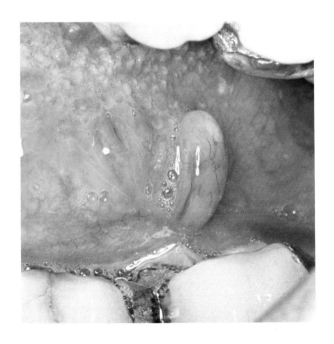

Black hairy tongue

Black hairy tongue (lingua villosa nigra) is the term applied to an extraordinary overgrowth of the filiform papillae giving the tongue a superficial semblance of hairiness. The condition is always found anterior to the terminal sulcus. The filiform papillae become elongated or thickened. The elongation may be due to a delay in the normal shedding of the horny layer of the filiform papillae, or the rate of formation of keratinized material may be increased. The individual filiform papillae may reach a length of 15–20 mm and 2 mm in diameter. In most cases, the affected area of the dorsum of the tongue appears as a mat. The color of the hairy tongue may vary from white to yellow, from greenish to bluish and, most commonly, from brown to black. It is therefore occasionally misleading to use the expression "black hairy tongue"; for these cases the term "hairy tongue" should be applied[104]. The pigmentation is due to overgrowth of chromogenic microorganisms. The pathogenesis of hairy tongue is still obscure. A considerable number of hairy tongue cases are idiopathic, as was the patient shown here, a 48-year-old woman who suddenly, without any demonstrable cause, discovered that her tongue was showing a black covering.

Hairy tongue

The patient pictured here suffers from an idiopathic hairy tongue. She is a 30-year-old woman who had been disturbed for a long time by an excessive overgrowth of the filiform papillae. In the picture it is possible to identify individual filiform papillae which are 6 to 7 mm long and heavily keratinized. It is characteristic that the "hairs" point to the lateral borders of the tongue. Understandably enough, the patient complained of a tickling sensation when the papillae touched the palatal mucosa. An idiopathic hairy tongue may quickly disappear or may persist for years. Apart from the idiopathic cases of hairy tongue, a number of factors are known to produce the condition, especially the use of antibiotics and corticosteroids. Other possible causes are the use of certain mouthwashes, e.g. hydrogen peroxide, poor oral hygiene, heavy smoking and gastrointestinal disorders. In the cases of hairy tongue produced by antibiotics it has been suggested that the drug alters the microbial flora, allowing an overgrowth of fungi. The many attempts at culturing these fungi have not produced uniform results. When treatment with antibiotics is discontinued, the hairy tongue may disappear within a few weeks.

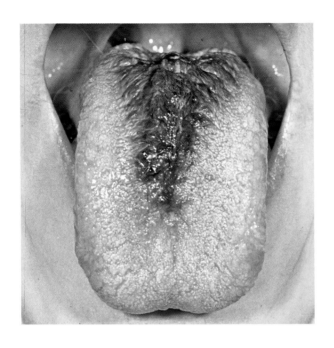

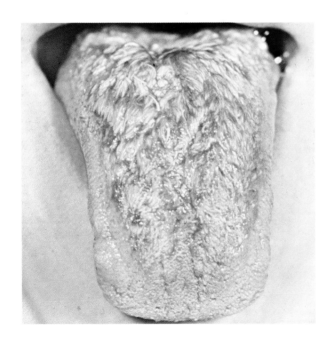

Plicated tongue

The plicated tongue is most often a developmental anomaly. It has several synonyms: "fissured tongue", "scrotal tongue", and "lingual dissecta". The prevalence of plicated tongue has been reported as 7 percent in an unselected Swedish population[24]. Among 6090 Iraqi schoolchildren plicated tongue was found in 2.6 percent[206]. The prevalence is much higher among mentally defective patients. The condition is found more frequently in older than in younger patients, thus raising doubts regarding its congenital nature. The plicated tongue is one of the signs of the Melkersson-Rosenthal syndrome (p. 158). Clinically, the plicae or fissures may present great variations in pattern. The most common pattern is one marked central fissure, anteroposteriorly, from which smaller fissures radiate laterally like the ribs in a leaf, as in the 39-year-old woman shown opposite. This pattern is demonstrated clearly when the patient stretches her tongue. Other patterns are the cerebriform and the transverse. The fissures may be relatively shallow, or they may be deep, in which case food debris will accumulate and result in inflammation. Twenty percent of plicated tongue patients will also have a geographic tongue[494].

Glossodynia

The terms glossodynia or glossalgia are used to describe a painful tongue and the term glossopyrosis for a burning sensation in the tongue. A burning sensation of the oral mucosa, especially the tongue, is not an uncommon complaint. Mainly postmenopausal women are affected. In a material of 292 patients in a general practice in England 5.1 percent had or had had a burning sensation of the mouth, the highest prevalence was found in the 40–49 year age group[47]. Among 100 diabetics and among 114 menopausal women the same investigator found prevalences of a burning sensation in 10 percent and 26 percent, respectively. In a German material of 72 patients with glossodynia, 76 percent were women with an average age of 60 years[231]. Patients with glossodynia can be divided into those who do not show any obvious pathologic changes and those with clinical changes of the tongue. The majority (about 75 percent) belongs to the first group, which presents a very difficult therapeutical problem. In some patients a reddening and loss of the keratinized layer of the filiform papillae on the tip of the tongue can be observed as in this 61-year-old woman illustrated. These changes are due to tongue-thrusting or tongue-pressure against the teeth or the palate.

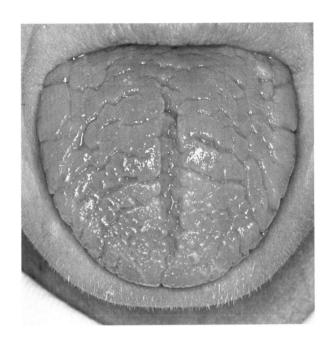

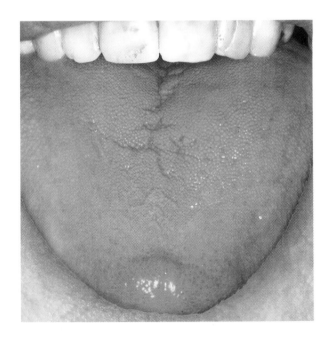

Crenated tongue

Impressions or indentations of the teeth observed at the lateral margin of the tongue are not rare phenomena. Because of the scalloped appearance, the condition is called crenated tongue. The indentation markins may have a different etiology. A great number of people suffer from an abnormal tongue pressure habit, and some from a tongue thrusting habit. In both habits the result is often impressions of the teeth on the tongue. The patient shown here is a 59-year-old woman who, for a long time, has had the habit of pressing the tongue hard against the teeth. As the mandibular incisor teeth were the site of attrition and thus had very sharp edges, the trauma exerted towards the tongue was more damaging than if the teeth had had smooth surfaces. A vicious circle was thus established. The trauma will cause an inflammation of the periphery of the tongue, leading to a slight macroglossia whereby the indentations become even more marked. Any enlargement of the tongue may become associated with lingual indentations from the teeth. Usually the macroglossia is caused by a systemic condition (acromegaly, p. 128; amyloidosis, p. 136), but any inflammatory involvement of the mouth may cause enlargement of the tongue.

Crohn's disease

Crohn's disease or regional enteritis is a chronic relapsing inflammatory, granulomatous disorder of unknown etiology, most often originating in the second and third decades of life. The disease produces a variety of abdominal signs and symptoms amongst other debilitating symptoms of malabsorption. In one material[48] of 100 patients, nine had oral manifestations of Crohn's disease. Another report[57] has analyzed 24 cases from the literature and found that only four patients were women, in contrast to the reported occurrence of Crohn's disease, which shows no sex predilection. Most frequently affected are (1) the buccal mucosa showing a cobblestone pattern, (2) the vestibule demonstrating linear, hyperplastic folds occasionally ulcerated as in the 16-year-old man shown here with Crohn's disease[487], and (3) the lips appearing diffusely swollen and indurated. A chronic granulomatous cheilitis may be associated with an asymptomatic Crohn's disease of the lower gastrointestinal tract[79]. A biopsy from the illustrated lesion showed small non-caseating epithelioid granulomas with Langhans type giant cells and lymphocytic infiltrate. It has been suggested that the oral lesions in patients with Crohn's disease might represent a local immunologic reaction to oral antigens[48].

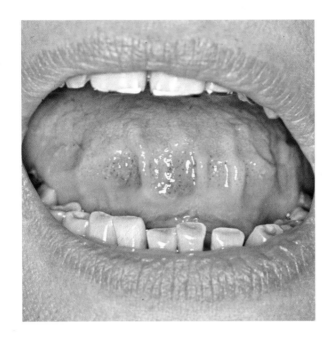

NON-INFECTIVE ENTERITIS

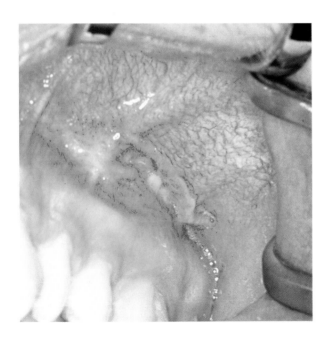

Uremia

Uremia is the clinical condition caused by the retention of urinary constituents in the blood. The characteristic symptoms of uremia are headache, vertigo, itching, nausea, convulsions, and eventually, coma. The patient's breath may have a urinous odor. Uremic patients may suffer from oral changes caused by the condition, but the frequency of oral involvement apparently is not very high. Subjective findings are an unpleasant taste and dryness of the mouth. Two types of oral manifestations are generally distinguishable: the most common type is erythematous, pseudomembranous uremic stomatitis, while the ulcerative type with crust formation is more rarely seen[265]. The patient pictured here, a 6-year-old girl, demonstrates the pseudomembranous type of uremic stomatitis. The blood urea level was 41 mmol/l at the time the picture was taken. Removal of the pseudomembranes exposes a dry, red, swollen mucosa. The stomatitis become manifest, when it occurs, after a few days of severe renal failure when the blood urea level exceeds 30 mmol/l. The oral bleeding tendency, often observed in uremic patients, is due to uremic thrombopathy. Uremic patients have an increased disposition to develop oral candidiasis[321].

COMPLICATION OF PREGNANCY, CHILDBIRTH, AND THE PUERPERIUM

Pregnancy gingivitis

The reported frequency of so-called "pregnancy gingivitis" varies between 30 and 100 percent, reflecting the diversity of opinion which exists. According to studies using well defined indices, a gingival change is noticeable from the second month of gestation, reaching a maximum in the eighth month. During the last month of gestation a definite decrease occurs. Furthermore, it has been found that the state of the gingiva after parturition is similar to that at the second month of pregnancy[345]. The prevalence of gingivitis in pregnancy seems to be offset to some degree by a concomitant decrease in debris accumulation[5]. Clinically, the gingival changes in pregnancy are characterized by a fiery red color of the marginal gingiva and interdental papillae. At the same time, the gingiva becomes enlarged, with the swelling mainly affecting the interdental papillae. The gingiva shows an increased tendency to bleed, and the patients sometimes experience slight pain. During pregnancy the gingival-periodontal index and the horizontal tooth mobility are increased[120]. The picture is of a 24-year-old woman in the sixth month of pregnancy. The gingival changes are characteristic, and they probably are aggravated by poor oral hygiene.

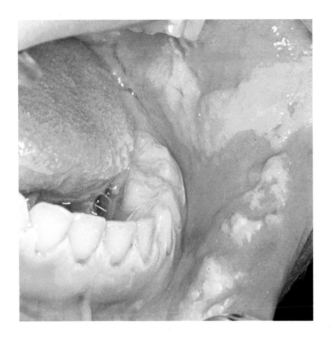

OTHER COMPLICATIONS OF PREGNANCY

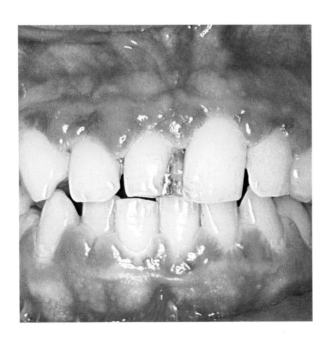

Pregnancy granuloma

Apart from the generalized gingival changes, pregnancy may also give rise to the formation of tumor-like growths, epulides, along the gingival margin. A number of terms have been suggested, such as "pregnancy tumor", "epulis gravidarum", and "pregnancy granuloma". The last-mentioned term is to be preferred, because the histologic structure is similar to the structure in pyogenic (telangiectatic) granuloma (p. 210). The reported frequency of pregnancy granuloma varies from 0 to 5 percent[555]. The granuloma occurs more frequently in the maxilla, favoring the vestibular aspect of the anterior region. It arises most often during the second trimester, occasionally earlier, and often shows rapid growth, although it seldom becomes larger than about 2 cm in diameter. After parturition, the granuloma begins to regress spontaneously and sometimes may disappear entirely. The pregnancy granuloma is mostly a pedunculated soft growth of interdental origin with a fiery red color and often with small fibrin-covered areas like those in the granuloma seen here, from a 31-year-old woman, in the eighth month of pregnancy. Pregnancy granulomas frequently will bleed readily when touched, and have a tendency to recur rapidly.

DISEASES OF THE SKIN AND SUBCUTANEOUS TISSUE

Pyostomatitis vegetans

In 1949 attention was called to the oral manifestations of Hallopeau's disorder, pyoderma vegetans, and the term pyostomatitis vegetans was suggested[359]. Besides skin lesions and ulcerative colitis, the pyostomatitis vegetans is characterized by oral lesions in the form of vegetations developed in areas of intense erythema. The vegetations, which are red in color, often have small raised yellow spots (pustules) from which a purulent material can be expressed. The oral manifestations are observed on the buccal mucosa, labial mucosa, palate, and gingiva. The illustrated patient is of a 63-year-old man who developed a painful pyostomatitis and dysphagia 3 months before admission to the hospital. There has been a great deal of confusion surrounding pyostomatitis vegetans, stemming form the uncertain and controversial etiology, the scarcity of patients, and particularly the variety of synonyms that have been applied to similar and possibly overlapping diseases[234]. The differential diagnoses center around pemphigus vegetans of Hallopeau and pemphigus vegetans of Neumann. Important in the distinction between pemphius vegetans (p. 240) and pyostomatitis vegetans is the presence of bowel disease and the lack of bullae in the latter[234].

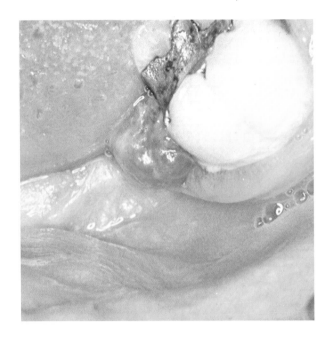

LOCAL INFECTIONS OF SKIN

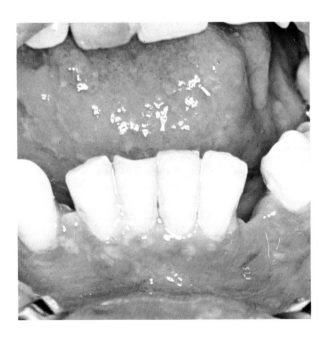

Acrodermatitis enteropathica

Acrodermatitis enteropathica, first recognized in 1942, is a rare genetically transmitted disease of infancy, following an autosomal recessive pattern. Its primary signs are: (1) skin lesions; (2) hair loss; (3) nail changes; and (4) diarrhea. The syndrome usually starts with small erythematous, moist skin eruptions which later become pustular, localized around the natural orifices. The perioral area is always affected in acrodermatitis enteropathica. Because of the pustular eruptions, weeping bilateral erosions at the angle of the mouth are often seen, at times with severe fissuring. Undoubtedly, a large number of children with the syndrome suffer from candidiasis. The buccal mucosa (less often the palate, gingiva, and tonsils) present reddish and white spots or edema with erosions, ulcerations, and desquamations. The patient illustrated is a 5-year-old girl whose brother also had the disease. She presented all the typical perioral and intraoral features of acrodermatitis enteropathica. Shortly after the second edition of this Atlas appeared in 1973 it was demonstrated that the disease is due to zinc deficiency[133]. Since then, many papers have reported on the successful treatment of acrodermatitis enteropathica with zinc supplements[534].

Allergic contact stomatitis due to acrylic denture material

It is generally accepted that allergic reactions to denture base materials are very rare[399]. The majority of complaints and palatal mucosal reactions to dentures belong to the type called "denture stomatitis", a chronic atrophic candidiasis (p. 62). Allergic reaction to dental rubber as denture base material has been reported, but this material is very seldom used in modern dental practice. The denture base material used today consists mostly of acrylic resins supplied in the form of a liquid (methylmetacrylate), the monomer, and a powder (polymethylmethacrylate), the polymer. Mixing these together and heating the dough causes the mixture to harden. Depending on the processing, varying amounts of residual monomer may be present in the denture. Usually, the monomer is regarded as the constituent most likely to sensitize the patient, but recently it has been questioned whether the allergic reactions are really due to the monomer. It has been suggested that the denture base material may acquire antigenic properties by continuous absorption of sensitizing agents[561]. The patient shown here is a 50-year-old woman who developed a fiery red stomatitis and skin reactions after having an acrylic denture inserted. The skin patch test was positive for the denture material.

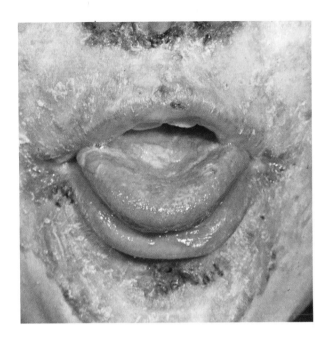

CONTACT DERMATITIS

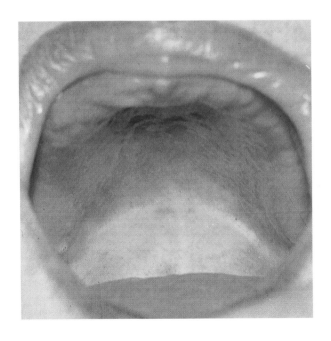

Allergic contact stomatitis due to toothpaste aromatics

Reactions to chemical contact allergens in the mouth, especially tooth-pastes, are rare due to (1) the rapid dispersal and absorption of allergens through the well-vascularized mucosa, (2) a short period of contact between ingredients and the oral mucosa, and (3) dilution and removal of potential allergens by saliva[187]. Among the agents causing an allergic reaction in the oral mucosa should be mentioned various metals (cobalt, nickel, silver and mercury), mouthwashes, denture adhesives, chewing gum, and lipstick. An unusual, allergic reaction was observed in the 38-year-old woman shown here[251]. After changing to a modification of a toothpaste, which had been marketed for a long time, the patient developed a diffuse, fiery red gingivitis and an erythema of the vestibular mucosa. Furthermore, a cheilitis was present. Earlier the patient had tolerated an ordinary toothpaste of the same brand, but an analysis showed that the new toothpaste contained oil of spearmint, carvone, and anethole which caused the allergic reaction of the patient. A symptom complex consisting of cheilitis, glossitis, and gingivitis has been described as an allergic gingivostomatitis due to chewing gum[297].

Allergic stomatitis due to eugenol

Eugenol, 4-allyl-2-methoxyphenol, is an old remedy which has been used for many years in every dental office. First of all as part of the zinc-oxide-eugenol temporary cavity dressing, but also as part of a gingivectomy pack. Furthermore, eugenol may be applied to gauze and placed in dry sockets to alleviate pain. Allergic contact dermatitis due to eugenol has been reported among several dentists. The picture opposite illustrates, on the buccal mucosa of a 37-year-old woman, a contact stomatitis due to eugenol[42, 380]. Two weeks before admission the patient had the mandibular left first molar extracted. As the extraction caused considerable pain a piece of gauze wetted with eugenol was placed in the socket and the patient received a bottle with eugenol and gauze and instructions on how to change the gauze daily. After 9 days the patient experienced an itching and burning sensation of the oral mucosa in the left side of the mouth. Clinically, numerous small, fibrin-covered ulcerations on an erythematous mucous membrane were found on the buccal mucosa, left side of the tongue and alveolar ridge. Skin patch tests with eugenol and balsam of Peru were positive. After withdrawal of the eugenol treatment, the ulcerations disappeared in the course of 3 days.

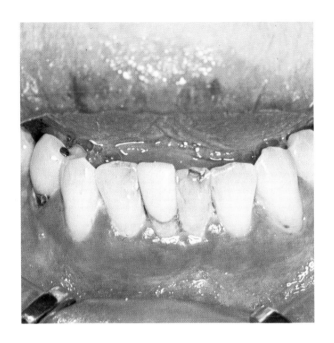

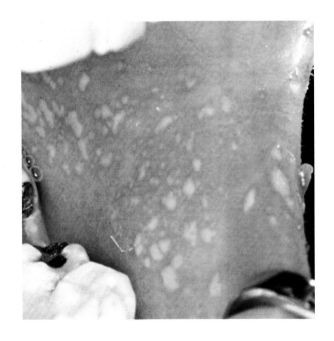

Allergic contact stomatitis due to propolis

Propolis is the name for bee glue, a dark yellowish-brown resinous substance with strong adhesive properties. Mixed with wax, it is used by bees to seal up crevices in the hives, to smooth the surfaces and to protect the entrance from intruders[584]. It is collected by honeybees from the resinous exudations of plants and trees, especially poplar trees. Usually, propolis contains wax 30 percent, resins and balsams 55 percent, essential oils 10 percent, pollen 5 percent, and cinnamic alcohol, minerals and flavorids[584]. Beekeeper's dermatitis due to propolis is well known. In the last decades there has been an increasing use of propolis preparations in the form of tablets, solid propolis, powder, ointment and cosmetic creams because of its presumed healing properties. The first examples of contact dermatitis and stomatitis due to propolis, taken for mental depression and gingivitis, have now been reported[584]. The patient shown here is a 74-year-old woman who applied solid propolis in the mandibular groove for a sore throat. After a few days, superficial ulcerations appeared around the sublingual caruncula and in the groove. When the patient stopped the application of propolis, the lesions disappeared.

Lesion related to amalgam restoration

So-called electrogalvanically induced leukoplakias were first described[569] in 1933. Later, a study has demonstrated a remarkable improvement of the mucasal lesions when harmfully high potentials were removed[269]. In a combined Danish-Hungarian study of 1454 patients with either leukoplakia or lichen planus, where 32 patients showed oral mucosal lesions which could be attributed to electrogalvanism, it was suggested to use the term "electrogalvanically induced oral white lesions"[37]. This concept was emphasized in the report from an international seminar on leukoplakia and the term suggested was "lesions associated with dental restorations". The term "electrogalvanic" has been abandoned as it has not been proven that such lesions are due to differences in an electric potential. More likely, the mucosal changes may be due to the effect of corrosion products from amalgam fillings or from plaques accumulated on the corroded surface of the filling. The picture illustrate a 58-year-old woman with a white patch on the right buccal mucosa in close relation to a gingival amalgam filling in the first molar. The filling was replaced with plast and the picture to the right shows the disappearance of the white patch 3 months later. In such cases a contact allergy to mercury compounds have been found[330].

234

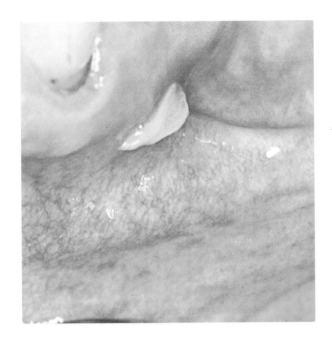

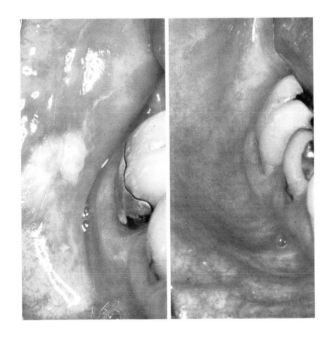

Allergic contact stomatitis due to gold inlay

Allergic reactions to metallic gold are rare and allergic contact stomatitis due to either gold dentures, gold crowns or gold inlays[201]. The first case of allergic contact stomatitis to gold was reported in 1970. After that time about 10 more cases have been published in the literature[257]. Although gold is a rather inert metal, the oral environment is moist and may permit slow dissolution of elemental gold into gold salts capable of provoking a reaction[593]. The oral mucosal reaction should be followed by a patch test. However, it should be pointed out that gold chloride commonly used for skin patch testing can easily give false positive reactions[201]. On the other hand, cases are on hand where the skin patch test has been negative, but an intraoral provocation test has been positive. The oral manifestations reported on earlier have consisted in erythema of the oral mucosa occasionally with petechiae and ulcerations. The illustrations shows a superficial ulceration of the labial mucosa in a 63-year-old man. When the mouth was closed the ulceration was in direct contact with gingival gold inlay in the maxillary right canine. The skin patch test for gold chloride was negative. The gold inlay was removed and replaced by a plast filling. After an observation period of 7 weeks the lesion had healed.

Dermatitis herpetiformis

The skin disease dermatitis herpetiformis, occasionally called Duhring's disease, is a rare, benign condition associated with a gluten-sensitive enteropathy. Immunopathologic studies have revealed deposits of mainly immunoglobulin IgA at the epithelial-connective tissue junction[114] and the presence of circulating anti-gliadin antibodies (gliadin is the active component of wheat gluten)[545]. It is characterized by the appearance of crops of blisters which may be preceded by erythematous patches. The blisters resemble herpetic lesions, as the name of the disease implies, and they appear especially on the trunk and limbs. Oral manifestations may be observed, although rarely. In most cases the oral lesions will appear after the skin affection. They may be seen in all areas of the oral mucosa, although the gingiva rarely is involved. The lesions consist of small, circular vesicles, which soon rupture, leaving fibrin-covered, superficial erosions. Some of the lesions may resemble aphthous ulcerations[479], and hyperkeratotic areas also are seen. The case illustrated, a 65-year-old man, demonstrates small vesicles, indicated by arrows, on an erythematous background. Development of pyogenic granuloma in the oral mucosa as a complication of dermatitis herpetiformis has been reported.

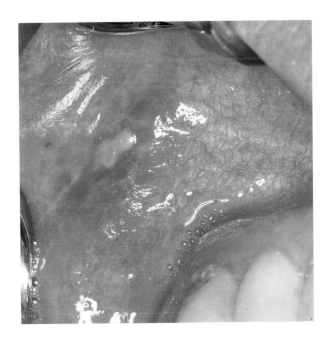

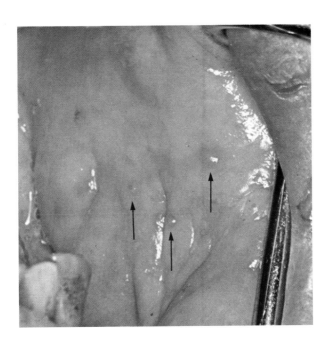

Pemphigus vulgaris

Pemphigus includes four types: pemphigus vulgaris, pemphigus vegetans, pemphigus foliaceus, and pemphigus erythematosus. An epidemiologic study among Jews in the Jerusalem area revealed an annual incidence rate of 1.6 per 100,000 population. Women were affected more than men and older persons (over 40 years) more than younger ones[320, 433]. Pemphigus is most likely an autoimmune disorder with IgG present at the cell periphery of basal and spinous cells as a reaction to an antigen located to the surface of these cells[129, 236]. Large bullae in all shapes appear on the skin; these bullae rupture easily and leave denuded areas. The natural course of pemphigus vulgaris was fatal until the introduction of steroid therapy. In the Jerusalem study, the oral mucosa was the sole initial site in 56 percent of the patients, while 88 percent of the cases have shown primary lesions of the oral mucosa alone or combined with other sites. Because of the humid environment and trauma, the bullae of the oral mucosa will rupture shortly after formation, leaving a nonspecific ulceration, making a correct diagnosis difficult[186]. An attempt has been made to classify oral lesions according to severity[249]. The picture illustrates a small intact bulla on the soft palate of a 48-year-old woman with pemphigus vulgaris.

Pemphigus vulgaris

The oral involvement is severe and very disturbing to the patients. As in the skin, bullae may not form, but the oral epithelium merely slides off as a result of the acantholysis occurring inside the epithelium. In this way large areas of the oral mucosa may become involved. Often epithelial tags are seen at the border of the superficial ulcerations. This is exemplified in the illustration opposite. It shows extensive fibrin-covered ulcerations on the buccal mucosa of a 34-year-old man. Any part of the oral mucosa may be affected in pemphigus vulgaris, although areas of trauma are more commonly affected. There appears to be a predilection for lesions to occur more frequently on buccal mucosa, palatal and gingival sites[618]. The fact that oral lesions often precede skin lesions will inevitably lead to a delay in establishing the proper diagnosis. This has been shown in a study where there was a 7-months' duration between onset and correct diagnosis. Pemphigus vulgaris rarely tend to have a sudden onset with severe and widespread lesions[320]. The rarer forms of pemphigus, the foliaceus and erythematous types, are believed not to have oral manifestations.

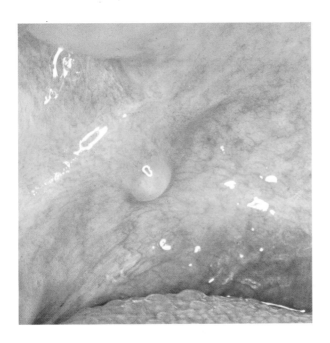

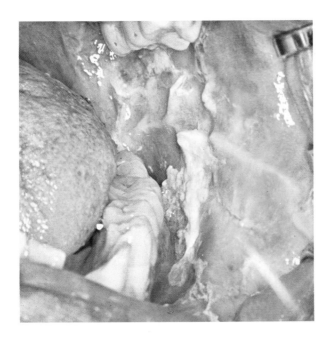

239

Pemphigus vegetans

Pemphigus vegetans is considered to be a milder form of pemphigus vulgaris and is characterized by the occurrence of fungoid vegetations which form on the erosions after the bullae have ruptured. The tendency to bulla formation is, however, less than in pemphigus vulgaris. The areas must frequently affected are the axillae and groin, the genitalia, the extremities, and the scalp. Like pemphigus vulgaris, the vegetans type begins, in more than half of the cases, in the oral cavity, often months before the skin lesions appear. Patients first exhibiting cutaneous lesions will ultimately develop oral manifestations[327]. The corners of the mouth are favored sites for pemphigus vegetans. All areas of the oral mucosa may be affected, mostly in the form of whitish, serpiginous lesions. Vegetating masses are not always found in the oral mucosa; the patient shown here, however, illustrates such a manifestation. This was a 71-year-old woman who had had pemphigus for 1 year. In the posterior part of the alveolar ridge, the buccal groove and buccal mucosa vegetating masses are seen. The whitish color indicates a hyperkeratosis, a change often observed after healing of bullae in the oral mucosa.

Benign mucous membrane pemphigoid

Pemphigoid is subdivided into bullous pemphigoid and benign mucous membrane pemphigoid both characterized by a subepithelial bulla formation and by identical oral lesions. Most, but not all, patients with both types of pemphigoid have deposition of gammaglobulins at the epithelial-connective tissue junction, and most patients with bullous pemphigoid have circulating antibodies against a basement membrane zone antigen[236]. In patients with benign mucous membrane pemphigoid only some will have such circulating antibodies[130]. Bullous pemphigoid affects is dominated by skin affections, with only 39 percent of patients exhibiting oral manifestations[320]. The benign mucous membrane pemphigoid primarily affects women and almost invariably involves the oral mucosa[517]. Oral manifestations were the only sign of the disease, irrespective of its duration. The initial oral changes consist of a yellow or hemorrhagic bulla originating on an erythematous background. Because of the moist environment, the bullae burst, leaving a fibrin-covered ulceration. The favored oral locations are the palate, the buccal mucosa, the gingiva, and the alveolar ridge. The illustration is from a 67-year-old woman with a typical lesion on the palate.

240

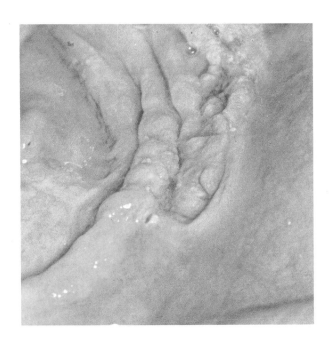

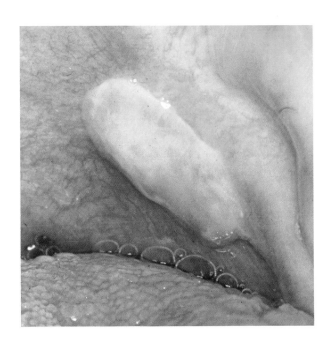

Benign mucous membrane pemphigoid

To some authors the most characteristic aspect of mucous membrane pemphigoid is a desquamative gingivitis, as in the 52-year-old woman shown opposite. The first indication of this systemic disease was the gingival changes. The gingiva is fiery red and tags of loose epithelium can be identified in several areas. Nowadays it is generally agreed that the majority of the cases of desquamative gingivitis are either mucous membrane pemphigoid or erosive lichen planus (p. 252). The oral lesions in pemphigoid are aggravated by the presence of local irritants such as calculus, ill-fitting crowns and bridgework, and dentures. It is interesting to note, however, that well-functioning full upper dentures seem to protect the palatal mucosa. About 65 percent of the patients with pemphigoid will have their first manifestation of the disease in the oral mucosa. The bullae in mucous membrane pemphigoid may develop rapidly and may remain for 2 or 3 days before rupturing. A follow-up of 26 patients with pemphigoid revealed intraoral scarring at the sites of earlier pemphigoid lesions. As the ocular and pharyngeal changes are quite severe and followed by scars, the term cicatricial mucosal pemphigoid has been suggested[197]. Oral pemphigoid may resemble oral pemphigus.

Erythema multiforme exudativum

The most outstanding features of erythema multiforme exudativum (syn. Stevens-Johnson syndrome, Fiessinger-Rendu syndrome, and ectodermosis pluriorificialis) are stomatitis, conjunctivitis, balanitis, and skin lesions. The disease, seen primarily in young adults and more frequently in men, has an acute onset, and runs a selflimited course from one to several weeks. It is often preceded by an upper respiratory infection, and fever frequently is present. The cutaneous lesions vary from small papules to extensive lesions and often have an iris-like shape with a central indentation. The frequency of oral manifestations in erythema multiforme exudativum may vary from about 40 to 100 percent. Very characteristic is extensive crust formation on the lips. The illustration opposite, of a 25-year-old Negro, shows iris-like papules on the labial mucosa and crust formation on the vermilion border. The crust formation can be helpful in making the diagnosis. The oral lesions, which have been reported to go through the following stages: macular, bullous, sloughing, pseudomembranous, and healing, are seen also on the buccal and gingival mucosa, tongue, and hard and soft palate.

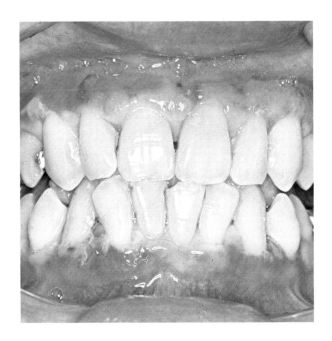

ERYTHEMATOUS CONDITIONS

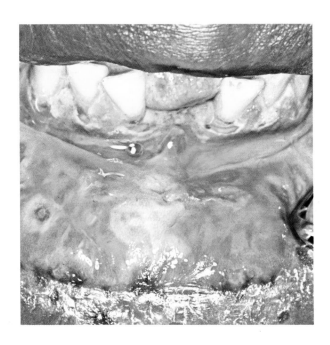

Erythema multiforme exudativum

Because of the humid environment and movements of the mucosal tissues during mastication, the oral lesions are not so well-defined as the cutaneous ones. The initial stage in the development of the oral lesion is a small erythematous plaque which is soon followed by a vesicle or bulla; these bullae or vesicles, however, are only infrequently observed as they are. The ruptured vesicles or bullae become confluent, forming shallow erosions covered by a necrotic exudate or pseudomembrane as seen in the 24-year-old man opposite. The lesions are susceptible to secondary infection, which may influence the clinical picture. Usually, erythema multiforme exudativum is recurrent. It may also occur as a disease located to the oral mucosa alone[339]. As to the etiology of erythema multiforme, a multitude of causative factors have been incriminated including a variety of bacterial, viral, and fungal infections, gastrointestinal upset, and allergy against drugs. The latter factor is more important than hitherto realized. In a material of 62 patients with a drug history oral mucosal involvement was found in thirty-one[205].

Discoid lupus erythematosus

Lupus erythematosus (LE) is an autoimmune disorder of unknown etiology usually divided into chronic discoid. LE and the acute (DLE) systemic type (SLE, p. 260). The discoid type is characterized by skin affections, especially on the skin of the nose and the malar eminences (butterfly pattern). The scalp, ears, and hands also may be affected. The cutaneous lesions consist of well-defined erythematous patches, adherent scaling, and follicular plugging. In addition, older lesions show atrophic scarring. Concerning the frequency of oral manifestations in all types of lupus erythematosus, the figures in the literature vary from 4 percent to 25 percent[482]. The four important elements of oral discoid lesions are: (1) a central atrophic area with (2) small, white dots (keratinized horn plugs) and a slightly elevated border zone of (3) irradiating white (keratinized) striae, and (4) telangiectasia[482]. These features can be seen in the illustration opposite, which is from a 45-year-old man. The white areas are keratinized. Isolated oral lesions of DLE may exist without skin changes. Discoid lesions of the oral mucosa are infected by yeasts in about one half of the cases. Immunopathologic studies show deposits of immunoglobulins (Ig), complement (C) and fibrinogen at the basement membrane area[482].

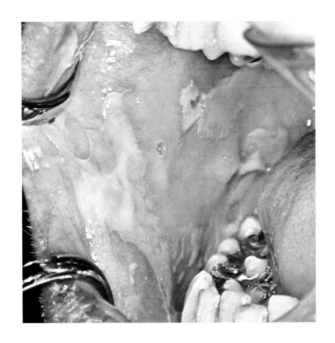

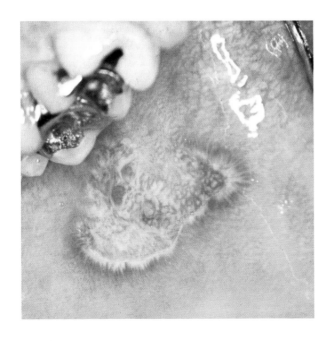

Discoid lupus erythematosus

A burning sensation from hot and spicy food and tenderness from tooth-brushing are the dominating symptoms[482]. The buccal mucosa is most often the seat of oral manifestations of discoid lupus erythematosus. Next in frequency are gingiva (alveolar process/ridge), labial mucosa, and vermilion border. When the vermilion border is affected, the first stage is characterized by a diffuse or localized erythema with a few telangiectasias. After some time an adherent, indurated keratotic scaling appears, and the fully developed lesion shows minute white dots. Lesions, localized to or involving the entire vermilion border may eventually extend onto the labial mucosa as well as the adjacent skin. The illustration opposite clearly shows these changes in a 35-year-old woman. The white dots represent what histologically is called horn plugs. After several years, the oral lesions may turn into leukoplakia-like white plaques. This change is apparently not associated with tobacco habits[482]. The atypical types of oral DLE may suggest several differential diagnostic possibilities. Some authors have described the development of cancer in discoid lupus erythematosus lesions located at the vermilion border, and it seems that men are more prone to develop cancer in oral lesions than are women.

Psoriasis vulgaris

Psoriasis vulgaris is a common, chronic, relapsing inflammatory skin disease characterized by rounded, circumscribed, erythematous, usually dry, scaling patches of a silvery-white color. The skin eruptions, which are most often symmetrical, have a predilection for the scalp, nails, elbows, and knees. The present author believes that there are four types of psoriatic oral lesions. The first type consists of minute, well-defined, gray to yellow-ish-white lesions which are round or oval. The white covering can be scraped off leaving a patchy, bleeding surface. The second type is characterized by whitish plaques with red areas on the oral mucosa[153]; these eruptions parallel those of skin[99]. The third type consists of a fiery red erythema of the oral mucosa mostly seen in the acute forms of psoriasis. The fourth type of oral lesion described in psoriasis is a geographic tongue (p. 216) which occurs more frequently among patients with psoriasis than without. The patient seen here is an 18-year-old boy who had had psoriasis for 2 months. He presented the typical picture of a geographic tongue. In a Finnish material of 200 patients with psoriasis 10 percent had changes of the oral mucosa suggestive of psoriasis. However, only four of the 20 biopsies showed changes typical of psoriasis[250].

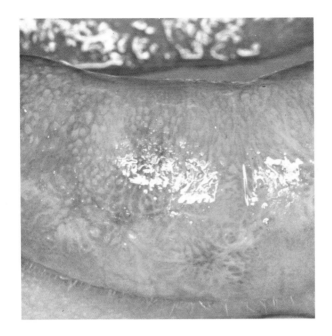

PSORIASIS

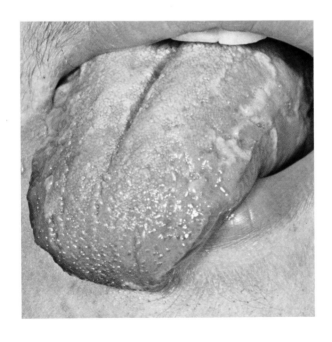

Pustular psoriasis

Extensive eruptions of minute sterile pustules may sometimes occur in the course of psoriasis, or may be the presenting symptom. The patients are usually seriously ill, and the condition as a whole is very resistant to treatment. Subungual pustules with shedding of the nails are common. Typical oral changes have been reported in patients with pustular psoriasis[495]. The manifestations comprise a variety of oral mucosa changes: diffuse mucous membrane inflammation, geographic tongue[314], red macular enanthema, foci of annulus migrans-like changes on gingiva, palate, and buccal and labial mucosa. Furthermore, the oral mucosa may be the seat of small, well-defined pustules. This change is exemplified in the illustration, which is from a 43-year-old woman who suffered from pustular psoriasis and whose nails also were severely affected. Besides the pustule in the left buccal mucosa, the illustration also reveals a plicated tongue (p. 222), which had several areas of lesions like those seen in geographic tongue. The pustules are caused by microabscesses in the epithelium. Pustule formation in the oral mucosa is rare. Pyostomatitis vegetans (p. 228) is another condition associated with the formation of oral pustules.

Reticular lichen planus

Lichen planus is a rather common inflammatory skin disease of unknown etiology characterized by the presence of small, flat, polygonal papules of a red-purple color. On the surface of the papules, delicate grayish-white lines can be observed, called Wickham's striae. The sites of predilection are the flexor surfaces of the body, e.g. the wrists, and the lesions are usually symmetric. The oral mucosa is often affected, but very few epidemiologic studies are available. In different geographic locations in India, where 85,000 persons were examined[425], the prevalence of oral lichen planus varied from .02 percent to 1.5 percent. In an unselected Swedish population a prevalence of 1.9 percent was found[24]. In Sweden there is a predominance of women in oral lichen planus patients. Also the oral lesions of lichen planus show great variation in clinical appearance. There are papular, reticular, plaque, atrophic, erosive (ulcerative) and bullous types. The most frequent type is the reticular pattern, which is illustrated here on the right buccal mucosa of a 67-year-old-woman. The characteristic findings are interlacing white lines, the Wickham's striae, which form a lattice-work or an annular arrangement. The buccal mucosa is the site most commonly involved.

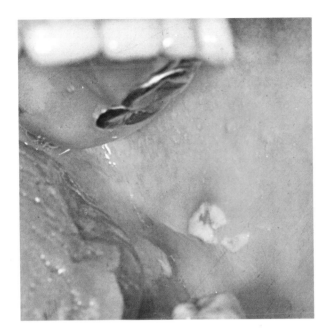

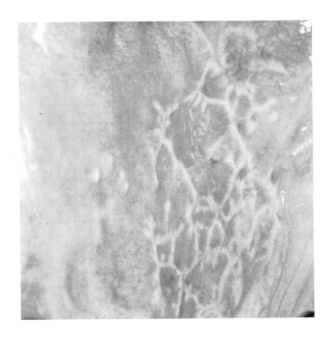

Plaque type of lichen planus

The picture opposite illustrates the plaque type on the left buccal mucosa in a 45-year-old man. In the posterior part of the buccal mucosa typical Wickham's striae are present. The same area is, however, characterized by white plaques similar to those which can be seen in a homogeneous leukoplakia. The presence, in the anterior part of the buccal mucosa, of very delicate keratinized striae, much finer than those of Wickham, indicates that the patient is enjoying tobacco to a considerable extent (p. 190). On questioning, the patient said that he, in fact, was smoking 25 cheroots daily. For the plaque type, found in 51 percent among 611 Danes with oral lichen planus, it has been demonstrated[393] that daily smokers showed significantly lower prevalences of reticular and atrophic types and a significantly higher prevalence of the plaque type. It is suggested that these findings depend on a mechanism whereby original atrophic and reticular types of lesions are altered into the plaque type of lesion under the influence of smoking. The question arises whether the plaque type of lesion can be regarded as leukoplakia which has been superimposed on the oral mucosa affected by lichen planus.

Atrophic lichen planus

Previously it was believed that oral lichen planus occurred when skin lesions were present. A number of studies, however, demonstrated that oral lichen planus may occur without any skin lesion[393]. In the Copenhagen material comprising 611 cases, skin lesions were present in only 32 percent. In one-third of these patients the oral lesions occurred simultaneously. The patient seen here, a 57-year-old woman, has a characteristic example of an atrophic lichen planus located on the left buccal mucosa. The dominant clinical feature is a reddening of the mucosa, caused by an atrophy of the epithelium. At the border of the red area, whitish Wickham's striae are observed. A gingival location of atrophic lichen planus, especially if the epithelium is ruptured, may have features similar to what has been called a desquamative gingivitis, but which is a nonspecific gingival manifestation of several systemic disturbances. Histologically, the atrophic type is characterized by a marked atrophy of the epithelium. As in all types of oral lichen planus there is a subepithelial lymphocytic infiltration with liquefaction degeneration of the basal layers. The lymphocytes have been shown to be predominantly T-lymphocytes[455]. There is a "sawtooth" appearance of the rete ridges.

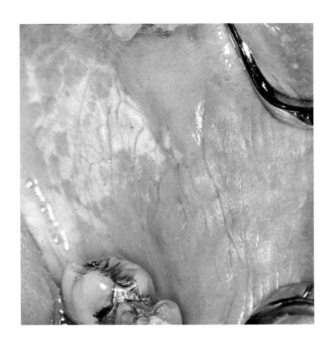

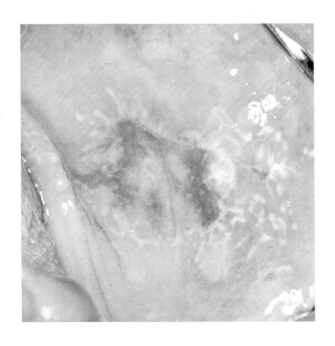

Erosive (ulcerative) lichen planus

Lesions of the atrophic type of oral lichen planus may ulcerate, whereby an erosive or ulcerative type is formed. This type accounts for about 7 percent of all oral lichen planus cases in the Copenhagen material[393]. Distinguishing between a minor and a major erosive type[567] has been suggested. The minor type is characterized by shallow ulcerations of the oral mucosa, often associated with milky-white areas of non-erosive lichen planus. The pain caused by the minor type is variable, but in most cases there is a considerable degree of discomfort. The major erosive type is much rarer than the minor type. In one series in England it made up for 7 percent of all oral lichen planus cases[569]. The predominant feature is widespread ulceration of the mucosa, most markedly the tongue. This is seen in the illustration opposite, of a 55-year-old woman. The ulceration may involve the entire dorsum of the tongue. The onset is rapid and there are always very disturbing subjective symptoms. In some patients presenting drug-induced stomatitis or contact stomatitis the lesions may have a lichenoid appearance. It has been suggested[342] that drugs that are known to induce lichenoid responses act as agents which amplify a disorder predating the use of the drug.

Bullous lichen planus

The bullous type of oral lichen planus is rare. The bullae may vary in size from a few milimeters up to several centimeters. Because of the moist environment in the oral cavity, the bullae will burst soon after their formation, leaving an ulcerated surface. The bullae probably are caused by edema in the connective tissue and a defect in the basement membrane. The patient seen here, a 34-year-old man, presented an intact small bulla on the palate. Close to the bulla there are reticular Wickham's striae. Many theories have been suggested to explain the etiology of lichen planus: (1) a bacterial origin, (2) a viral origin, and (3) a nervous or neurogenic theory. Recent investigators[52] suggest that aggregations of T-lymphocytes are responsible for the cytotoxic processes which occur within the squamous epithelium in oral lichen planus. The immunologic reaction possibly is related to antigenic changes of epithelial cell surfaces[259]. Other studies[523] suggest that patients with oral lichen planus may have a generalized immunologic disorder in which humoral immunity is disturbed. Two studies have demonstrated that oral lichen planus patients show (1) a higher correlation with delayed hypersensitivity to dental materials than a control population[173], and (2) a high frequency of contact allergy to mercury[185].

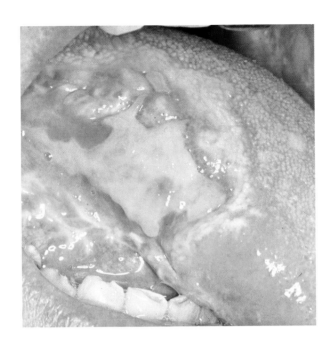

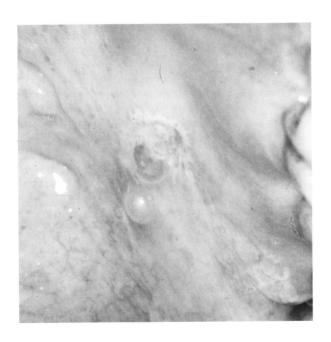

Malignant transformation in oral lichen planus

In the past oral lichen planus was regarded as a completely innocuous condition, but in the last couple of decades it has been vividly discussed whether lichen planus is a precancerous condition. Some investigators[310, 510] feel that the development of a squamous cell carcinoma within an area of histologically identified oral lichen planus does not conclusively substantiate a cause and effect relationship. One of the reasons why some American investigators have not been able to demonstrate the precancerous nature of oral lichen planus may be lack of follow-up studies to demonstrate the relationship between oral lichen planus and cancer. Other American investigators have concluded that oral lichen planus should be considered a premalignant condition in which incidence of transformation approaches that of oral leukoplakia yet clearly distinctive from that disease with regard to age and sex distribution[350]. It has been postulated[14], that most of the carcinomas to have arisen in oral lichen planus had done so from atrophic or erosive lesions. An exemption may be the patient illustrated opposite. In 1969 the 67-year-old woman was examined and a diagnosis of reticular lichen planus made on the lesion in the left buccal mucosa. At the time of examination she smoked two cheroots daily.

Malignant transformation in oral lichen planus

Twelve years after the patient, illustrated on the top of the opposite page, was examined first time, she returned with an ulceration in the posterior part of the left buccal mucosa. The ulceration had the characteristics of a carcinoma including indurated margins and a biopsy showed a squamous cell carcinoma. One investigator[567] has found that a carcinoma developed in an oral lichen planus following an intermediate period in which the lesion transformed into a speckled leukoplakia. Another study[229] followed two patients with oral lichen planus and found it changed into candidal leukoplakia with subsequent malignant transformation. Dorsum of the tongue which rarely is the seat of carcinoma has been reported affected by a carcinoma developing in an oral lichen planus in a number of cases[106, 436]. In a recent Dutch-Hungarian study of 100 cases of oral lichen planus it was found that in approximately 25 percent moderate or at least mild epithelial dysplasia was observed[139]. It is interesting to compare these findings with a statement from another Hungarian study that oral lichen planus is not a precancerous condition[316].

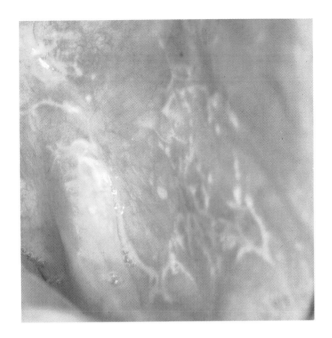

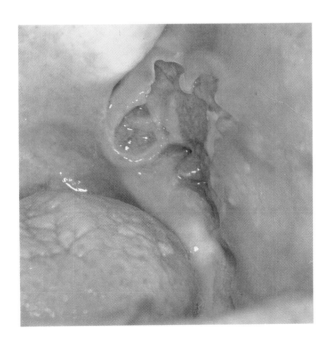

Erythroplakia associated with lichen planus

Usually it is stated that the atrophic and erosive types of lichen planus are the ones most likely to turn malignant. The question naturally arise: have all these cases of "atrophic" lichen planus been the true atrophic type or have they been erythroplakias? The author believes that erythroplakias may have been erroneously diagnosed as atrophic lichen planus cases in the past because erythroplakia has not been identified as a dangerous premalignant lesion *per se* for a very long time. In a material of 740 patients with oral lichen planus eight patients were found with a sharply demarcated, slightly depressed erythroplakic area[260]. The histologic examination of the biopsies from the eight erythroplakias showed epithelial dysplasia in seven cases. In addition, two of the lesions revealed a squamous cell carcinoma. One of the patients without carcinoma, a 75-year-old woman, is illustrated opposite. At the first examination a biopsy from the erythroplakia on the right buccal mucosa showed a mild epithelial dysplasia. The patient was followed every third month. After 3 years a papillomatous growth developed at the anterior part of the erythroplakia. Two years later proliferations of the mandibular gingiva in the front were removed and the histologic diagnosis was squamous cell carcinoma.

Keratoacanthoma

Keratoacanthoma is a not too rare benign cutaneous lesion which is believed to arise from hair follicles. The lesion is most frequently observed between 50 and 70 years of age, with a male:female ratio 3:1 and largely confined to Caucasians[496]. In the past the lesion often has been diagnosed as a squamous cell carcinoma. It is well-circumscribed, slightly elevated with crateriform excavation centrally, and slightly indurated borders, but there are no signs of infiltration. The etiology of keratoacanthoma is unknown, although some factors, like chemical carcinogens, immunosuppressive drugs, and sunlight, may play an etiologic role. The lesion may spontaneously regress and is easily cured by simple excision or curettage. Based upon a literature review 65 cases of lip keratoacanthomas have been analyzed[31]. Their age was significantly lower than for lesions on the skin. As there are no hairs on the vermilion border, it could be assumed that the keratoacanthoma has originated from sebaceous glands, which often are present in the area or just from the surface epithelium[172]. The picture illustrates a keratoacanthoma on the lower vermilion border in a 29-year-old man. The lesion, in a solitary form, may also occur intraorally.

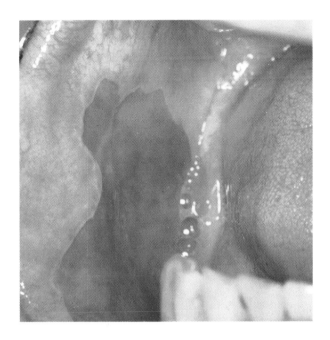

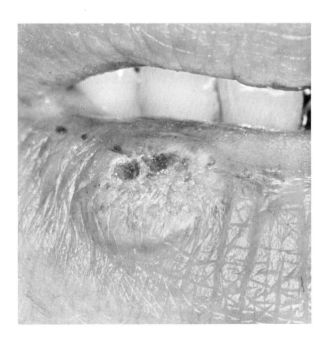

Malignant acanthosis nigricans

Acanthosis nigricans is defined as a rare cutaneous disorder characterized by hyperkeratosis and pigmentation, which occurs as an apparently isolated developmental defect[155]. One variant is the malignant acanthosis nigricans where involvement of the skin, in the form of hyperpigmented, hyperkeratotic verrucosities, may precede, accompany or follow the detection of a cancer, usually an adenocarcinoma. The skin changes are especially found in the axillae, the back and sides of the neck, the anogenital region, and the groins. Oral manifestations may be present in 30–40 percent[214]. Although oral changes often are mentioned the descriptions usually are meagre. One study has especially dealt with the characteristic oral manifestations, clinically as well as histologically[36, 385]. The illustration opposite, of a 64-year-old man, demonstrates typical changes at the left labial commissure, which is the seat of fungiform growths. The buccal mucosa presents a marked leukoedema. The contralateral commissure, the tongue and palate also were affected in a similar way. At the time of oral examination no malignancy could be demonstrated. However, after 1 year the patient developed an adenocarcinoma in the right lung. Other patients with malignant acanthosis nigricans may show a thickening of the labial mucosa and the vermilion border with a papillomatous pattern.

Actinic elastosis (cheilitis)

The condition illustrated opposite is seen quite often in elderly men having had an outdoor occupation for many years. Previously the condition was called senile elastosis, because it most often is seen in old people, but the accepted term nowadays is actinic elastosis (keratosis) or actinic cheilitis as the distinction between these two entities may not always be very clear. The patient here is a 65-year-old man who has worked as a farmer for 30 years. His vermilion border is not as sharply defined as it is in individuals not having had an outdoor occupation. The vermilion border is the seat of a slight crust formation and has in some areas a whitish color, which is not a leukoplakia. The presence of crust may carry this patient into the group of actinic cheilitis. The inability of the vermilion border to be associated with leukoplakia is clearly illustrated in the patient seen on p. 192. The actinic elastosis (keratosis), which is the result of sun damage, is characterized by an atrophic epithelium caused by a transformation of the underlying collagenous tissue into an avascular elastotic tissue. Cancer of the vermillion border is often preceded by an actinic elastosis. In a material of 776 lip carcinomas, not less than 83 percent had actinic elastosis demonstrated histologically[56].

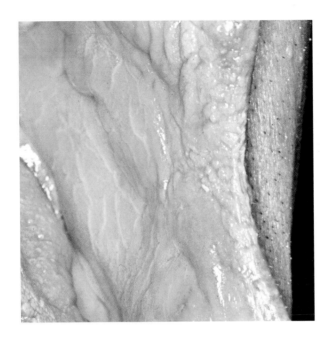

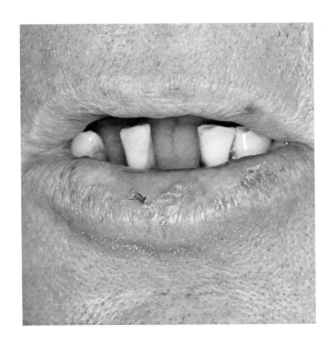

DISEASES OF THE MUSCULOSKELETAL SYSTEM AND CONNECTIVE TISSUE

Systemic lupus erythematosus

The oral manifestations of discoid lupus erythematosus are described elsewhere (p. 244). The acute or disseminated type of lupus erythematosus (SLE) is dominated by severe systemic symptoms of fever and pain in muscles and joints, as well as such blood changes as leukopenia and hypergammaglobulinemia. The cutaneous eruptions often begin in the face as a diffuse or patchy erythema and edema which, later on, spreads widely over the body. Sometimes, however, skin lesions do not appear at all. The disease, which now is considered to be an autoimmune disorder, often ends fatally. Oral manifestations in SLE have been reported to occur in 26–45 percent of patients[286, 572]. They present a varied picture. The outstanding oral changes are erythema and discoid lesions but rarely ulcerations[286]. White keratotic areas are not so frequently seen as in the discoid type. Other oral mucosal changes are edema and petechiae. The patient seen her, a 22-year-old woman, has suffered from affections of the skin, especially of the nose and cheeks, a butterfly exanthema, and paresthesia of the finger tips for a period of 3 years. Intraorally, she had multiple superficial, fibrin-covered ulcerations with focal spots of a slight hyperkeratosis. A biopsy confirmed the clinical suspicion of SLE. In one study specific immune deposits were found in all oral lesions examined[286].

Progressive systemic sclerosis

Progressive systemic sclerosis (PSS) also called diffuse scleroderma is a systemic disorder of connective tissue classified with autoimmune diseases like systemic lupus erythematosus, rheumatoid arthritis, and dermatomyositis. However, the role of immunologic abnormalities has not yet been firmly established. It occurs most often in the third and fourth decades of life, and women are more frequently affected than men. After an insiduous start the skin ends up by being very tight and firm. This can also be observed periorally, where furrows radiate from the atrophic vermilion border creating a socalled "tobacco pouch mouth". Subjectively, over 50 percent complain of xerostomia, limited opening, recurrent "mouth" sores and dysphagia[171]. The lips become immovable, making entry to the oral cavity difficult[219]. In patients with PSS the oral mucosa becomes pale and feels rigid upon palpation. The oral manifestations in PSS also include a shrinkage of the tongue in the late stage of the disease; it loses its mobility and papillary pattern as in the 73-year-old man shown here. Furthermore mastication is impaired. A striking dental finding in PSS is the widening of the periodontal membrane in 7–54 percent of the patients. Severe retraction of the gingiva has also been observed.

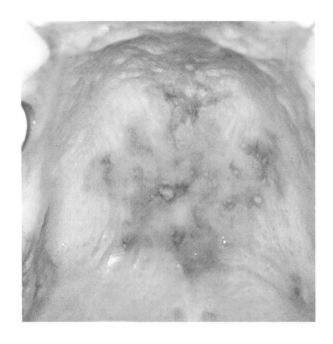

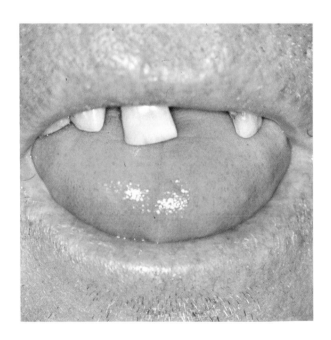

Sjögren's syndrome

In 1933, Sjögren described a group of patients exhibiting xerostomia, keratoconjunctivitis sicca, enlarged salivary glands and rheumatoid arthritis. When only oral and ocular manifestations are present, the term sicca syndrome is often used[349]. The syndrome occurs most frequently in women past menopause. A specific antibody to the cytoplasm in the salivary duct epithelium has been demonstrated in 75 percent of sera from patients with Sjögren's syndrome, one of many serum antibodies characterizing this autoimmune disorder[59, 349]. On clinical inspection, the oral mucosa is often so dry that the mirror used for the oral examination stick to the buccal mucosa. The color of the mucosa may vary from pale pink to fiery red, and small, sticky, ropy-like accumulations of saliva may be seen. The tongue will exhibit marked atrophy of the papillae, and later on the surface becomes smooth and lobulated, as in the illustration, of a 47-year-old woman. Focal sialadenitis in an adequate labial salivary gland biopsy is an objective criterion and a more disease-specific feature of Sjögren's syndrome than xerostomia or any others feature of salivary disease[134]. Patients with Sjögren's syndrome have an increased risk of developing lymphoma[489].

Dermatomyositis

Dermatomyositis is a clinical syndrome consisting of polymyositis associated with skin lesions. The disease is predominantly found in women and is of unknown etiology, although disordered immunologic mechanisms have been suggested[161]. The disease is characterized by muscle pain, loss of weight, weakness, fever, and arthralgia. The skin becomes the seat of violaceous erythema and edema, with a predilection for the eyelids, the malar area, and the dorsa of the hands. The edema which gives the skin a puffy consistency leaves a reticulated telangiectatic erythema when it subsides. The patients may die of respiratory or cardiovascular failure, or of debility and infection. The oral mucosa may be involved in dermatomyositis, although there is some disagreement as to how often this occurs. The oral mucosa may show erythema of a dark red or bluish color, probably caused by telangiectases[494]. Edema also may be found, especially on the gingiva as in the 8-year-old girl seen here. The marginal gingiva is fiery red and the capillaries are clearly seen on the background of the white dental enamel. The blackish color of the mandibular incisor is caused by treatment with Percy Howe's silver nitrate solution.

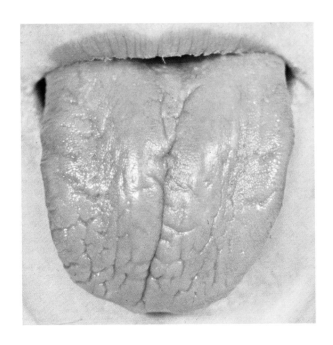

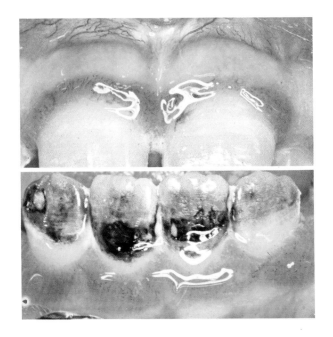

263

Tetralogy of Fallot

Congenital heart disease accounts for 1 to 2 percent of all organic heart disease in all age groups. Among the congenital forms, tetralogy of Fallot is one of the more frequent. It consists of (1) pulmonary stenosis, (2) a ventricular septal defect just below the aorta, (3) an aorta which overrides both the right and the left ventricles, and (4) hypertrophy of the right ventricle. Because of the intermixture of oxygenated and unoxygenated blood and the diminished flow of blood into the lungs due to the pulmonary stenosis, whereby the blood is not able to carry sufficient oxygen, the patients may exhibit cyanosis. Other changes due to the defects are clubbing of the fingers and a compensation polycythemia. The cyanosis, which may be present from birth, is obvious in the face and marked on the vermilion border. Also the oral mucous membrane may be darker than normal. The extremely cyanotic tongue seen here is from a 38-year-old man suffering from tetralogy of Fallot. The tongue is also plicated with a marked median fissure and a slight geographic tongue on the right side. High prevalences of plicated tongue and geographic tongue are in children with cyanotic congenital heart disease[230].

Tetralogy of Fallot

The gingival condition has been studied extensively in children with congenital heart disease. In most of these studies, tetralogy of Fallot has accounted for the largest group of the various anomalies. The color of the gingiva corresponds fairly closely to the general degree of cyanosis[218]. The cyanotic gingiva may be swollen as in the illustration, which is from an 11-year-old boy suffering from Fallot's tetralogy. Children with tetralogy will show a more marked periodontal destruction than healthy children in similar age groups. The cyanotic children will have deeper gingival pockets and will exhibit a lower level of oral hygiene and insufficient lip seal. When children with tetralogy of Fallot undergo corrective surgery, a postoperative clinical improvement of the gingival condition can be observed. Such an improvement has been demonstrated quantitatively by the use of stereoscopic photomicrography[196]. The number of subepithelial gingival blood vessels per mm² in patients with Fallot's tetralogy was significantly higher than in healthy subjects. After thoracic surgery, when the oxygen saturation showed normalized values, the number of gingival blood vessels decreased to normal.

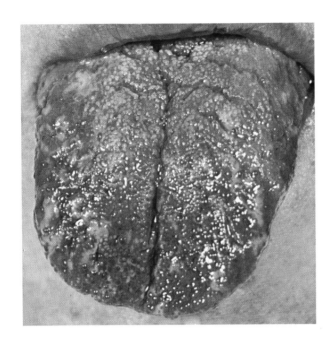

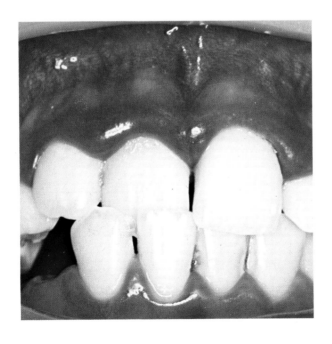

Cleft uvula

A cleft or bifid uvula is a minor manifestation of a more severe cleft of the palate. An epidemiologic survey of 7,837 students in Minnesota showed a 1.5 percent prevalence of cleft uvula[369]. In the survey uvula was classified into A: normal, B: bifurcated up to one fourth of its total length, C: bifurcated from one fourth to three fourths, and D: split from three fourths to its total length. Type B clefts had a prevalence of 1.2 percent, whereas C and D types had a 0.2 and 1.1 percent prevalence, respectively. The cleft uvula was slightly more common in men than in women. A genetic study was done on the same material, whereby it was demonstrated that 30 percent of the siblings of cleft uvula probands with parents simi-larly affected also had cleft uvula, indicating a transmission pattern of autosomal dominance with limited penetrance similar to that reported for isolated cleft palate. A survey in Minnesota of 635 Red Lake Chippewa Indian schoolchildren revealed a 10.2 percent prevalence of cleft uvula[108]. The relative prevalence of cleft uvula increased with increasing proportion of Indian ancestry. A survey from British Columbia revealed cleft uvula in 6.8 percent among Mongoloids and in 4.0 percent among Cau-casians[224]. The cleft uvula illustrated here was found in a 15-year-old boy.

Cleft lip

Cleft lip has been defined as a cleft extending into and through the alveolus as far as the incisive foramen. A combination of cleft lip and cleft palate is more common than isolated cleft lip. The incidence of cleft palate and cleft lip is about 1 per 1,000 live births of Caucasians, but isolated cleft lip is found in only 1 per 9,000 live births[532]. An increase in the incidence of cleft lip has been reported from 1938 to 1957 in Denmark[195]. In Australia, a decline in incidence of cleft lip with and without cleft palate has been linked to changes in birth rate[77]. Cleft lip results when the intimacy of contact between lateral nasal and medial nasal processes falls below a certain critical threshold, resulting in failure of fusion between the epithelia at the lower end of the nasal pit, and subsequent breakdown of the bridge joining the three processes[198]. Cleft lip with and without cleft palate appears to be caused by variable combinations of genetic and teratologic factors, depending for their effect on the time of embryogenesis at which they operate[77]. Cleft lip may be unilateral (80 percent), as in the 2-year-old girl seen here, or bilateral. When unilateral, the cleft is found on the left side in about two-thirds of the cases. There is a cleft palate more often with bilateral than with unilateral clefts of the lip.

266

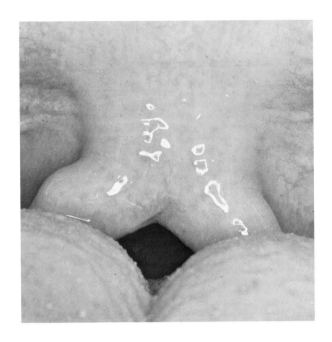

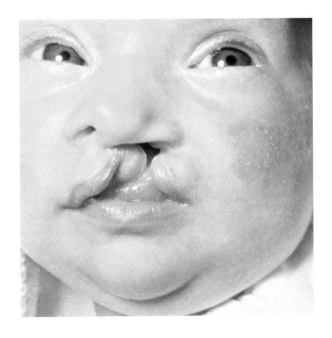

Ankyloglossia

Ankyloglossia or "tongue-tie" is due to an abnormally tight lingual frenulum, fibrous or muscular, which may bind the tongue to the floor of the mouth to varying degrees. This defect of the tongue may be either congenital or traumatic. The prevalence of congenital ankyloglossia varies from 0.04 percent to 6.8 percent. The ankyloglossia may cause deformities in the dental occlusion, especially spacing of the mandibular incisors and an open bite deformity, and may contribute to a periodontal lesion as in the 13-year-old boy shown here. Ankyloglossia has often been accused of causing speech defects. In a study of 1,000 children with disorders of speech, only four had seriously shortened frenums[364]. It can be reasonably presumed, therefore, that ankyloglossia plays only a minor role in the etiology of speech defects. A syndrome called "ankyloglossum superius syndrome" has been described where the tongue congenitally is attached to the hard palate or the maxillary alveolar ridge. Other defects in this syndrome are microglossia, hypodontia, and anomalies of the extremities[214].

Congenital lip pits

Congenital lip pits, also called congenital lip sinuses, are small depressions on the vermilion border, most often occurring as a symmetric pair, as in the 25-year-old man shown opposite. The condition is among the rarest of congenital anomalies with approximately 170 published cases. Rarely, the congenital lip pits may be unilateral, median, and bilateral asymmetric. The pits have been reported to occur on the labial mucosa in some cases. The fistula, which may be up to 3 mm in diameter, extends through the orbicularis oris muscles to a depth of 0.5 cm to 2.5 cm and communicates with the underlying salivary glands. Apart from the cosmetic handicap, the pits are annoying only when a viscid saliva comes out of the fistula. The most commonly accepted theory for the origin of the lip pits is that they are remnants of the lateral sulci of the lip during the fetal period. The pits are associated with cleft lip-cleft palate in 67 percent. The frequency of the syndrome has been estimated as 1:75,000 to 3:100,000 among Caucasians[107, 463]. Family histories can be explained adequately on the basis of autosomal dominant inheritance with variable expressivity of the trait. (Courtesy of Dr. I. SEWERIN, Copenhagen, Denmark).

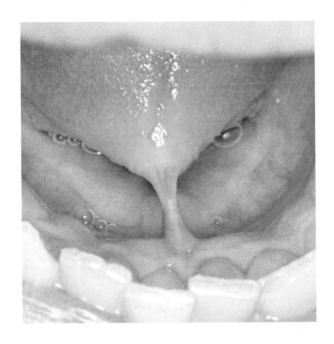

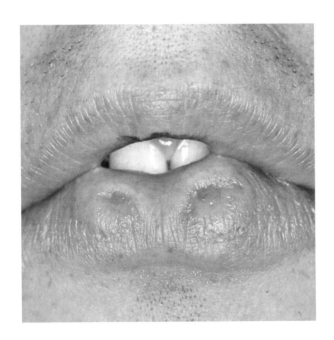

Fordyce's condition

Fordyce's condition or Fordyce's spots are names given to sebaceous glands occurring in the oral mucosa or in the vermilion border. The glands have a characteristic clinical appearance as small, well-defined, slightly elevated, yellowish or whitish granules which may be isolated or may occur in a confluent way as in the picture, which is from a 47-year-old man. They usually are seen in the buccal mucosa and upper vermilion border, with a symmetric distribution. The glands also may be found in the mucosa over the alveolar process and in the anterior pillar of the fauces. Large sebaceous glands are most often observed in the lower alveolobuccal sulcus. In adult Danes the prevalence is 80 percent for the vermilion border and 95 percent for oral sebaceous glands[506]. The prevalence is approximately the same in adult men and women. The extent of the glands is greater, the density higher, and the size larger in men than in women. Prevalence, extent, density, and size vary with age. The prevalence reaches a peak at 20–29 years of age. Size increases in men up to the age of 50–59. No function can be assigned to the glands, but the secretion may play a role of protection.

White sponge nevus

The anomaly to be described here has been reported under a variety of names: "white sponge nevus", "oral epithelia nevus", "familial white folded dysplasia of the mucous membranes", "developmental leukokeratosis", "nevus spongiosus albus mucosae", and "leukoedema exfoliativum mucosae oris". It is a congenital disturbance of the oral mucosa genetically transmitted by an autosomal dominant mode of inheritance[615] which manifests itself early in childhood and increases throughout life. The white sponge nevus usually is symptomless. The affected oral mucosa appears white or gray, thickened, deeply folded (almost scrotal), and spongy; the lesions are most often bilateral and symmetric. Younger people may display more pronounced lesions than older ones[38]. Although all areas of the oral mucosa may be affected, the characteristic features of the condition are best observed in the buccal mucosa, as in the illustration. This is a 35-year-old man who had been aware of his white sponge nevus since the age of 6 years. His father and brother are also affected. Some patients also exhibit lesions in the vaginal or rectal mucosa. The condition may show variations in intensity and may be mistaken for leukoplakia.

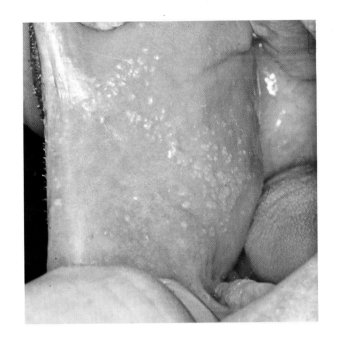

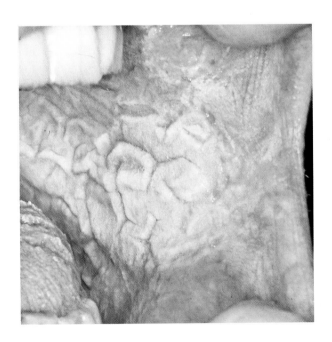

Nevus unius lateris

The condition to be described here is known also as ichthyosis hystrix and can be classified as an epidermal nevus. The patient seen here, a 26-year-old man, represents an extreme variant of a nevus unius lateris, as his entire left side is affected by the nevus, extending from the toes to the scalp, with a sharp demarcation at the healthy side. He also has characteristic oral manifestations. Apart from the tongue, the palate and the left buccal and labial mucosa are affected. The tongue is sharply divided into two halves by the nevus. The affected side is hypertrophic and characterized by loss of filiform papillae. When the lips are affected, the lesions are often condylomatous, mamillated or like flat papillomas, and the wart-like lesions may be rose, yellow, tan, dark brown, or gray[82]. The lesions of the buccal mucosa are often white or opalescent, occasionally exhibiting a spongy appearance. In the palate, a verrucous midline ridge may extend posteriorly over the hard and soft palate to a bifid uvula. When the gingiva is affected, large masses of verrucous lesions may cover part of the teeth.

Dyskeratosis congenita

This rare heritable disorder, also called "Zinsser-Engman-Cole syndrome", was originally described as reticular atrophy of the skin with pigmentation, dystrophy of the nails, and oral leukoplakia[539]. Later aplastic anemia, hypersplenism, and hyperhidrosis of the palms and soles were found also in other patients. A prominent reticulated hyperpigmentation of the skin is seen on the face, neck, and chest. In most cases the fingernails and toenails become dystrophic at about the age of puberty. The oral manifestations consist of crops of vesicles and bullae appearing on the oral mucosa, most frequently during the 5- to 7-year-old period. Because of moisture and maceration, they rupture early, leaving ulcerated areas and, after several attacks, the mucosa becomes atrophic and the tongue loses its papillae and appears smooth[214]. Eventually, the mucosa becomes thickened, fissured, and white (leukoplakic). The leukoplakias progress with increasing age[599]. All cases published previously have been in men, but the 27-year-old patient shown opposite is a woman. She had leukoplakic lesions on the palate and on the tongue, and the buccal mucosa appears slightly verrucous. Histologic examination of these lesions revealed hyperorthokeratotic changes.

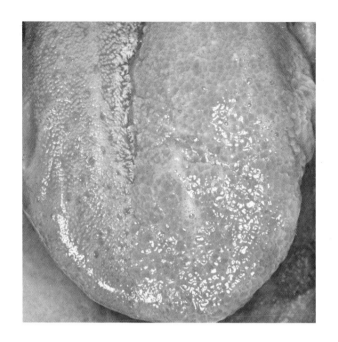

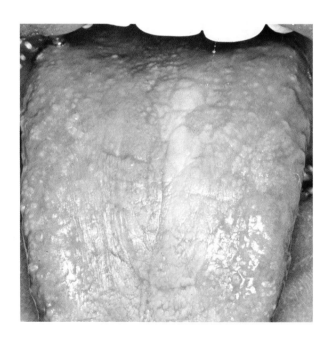

273

Dyskeratosis follicularis

This condition, which also has been reported under the names "Darier's disease" or "keratosis follicularis", is a rare skin disorder with a simple, dominant heredity[544] affecting both males and females. The skin lesions consist of multiple, hard, rough papules, often up to several millimeters in diameter and reddish in color. The lesions, which are heavily keratinized, ulcerate, coalesce, crust, and become verrucous and foul-smelling. They are not necessarily restricted to the follicles. The oral mucosa is affected in approximately 50 percent of the patients[544], but the degree of oral involvement does not necessarily run parallel with the degree of skin involvement[530]. The oral lesions are able to develop in the absence of the appendages seen in the skin, such as hairs and sweat glands. The oral elements, which may be seen especially on the gingiva, the tongue, and the palate, are small, rather flat coalescing papules, indicating that there is tendency for the papules to be restricted to keratinized areas of the oral mucosa. The patient seen here is a 49-year-old man who has a severe epidermal affection of dyskeratosis follicularis. Besides the palate, the tongue exhibits the same type of lesions.

Dystrophic epidermolysis bullosa

Epidermolysis bullosa is a rare condition characterized by bullous and vesicular eruptions of the skin and mucous membranes. The disease may occur in three types: simple, dystrophic, and lethal. The simple type is a mild form of the disease, and oral involvement is rare. The dystrophic type is inherited according to at least two patterns, autosomal dominant and recessive. The chief clinical feature of the dystrophic type, the formation of bullae, usually is manifested at or shortly after birth. The bullae arise at sites of pressure or trauma, but also may appear spontaneously. Upon healing, the bullae often are followed by keloidal scars. The dystrophic type will present oral manifestations in a considerable number of the cases. Most often the tongue seems to be affected, assuming a gray, smooth appearance and being thickened and deformed in some individuals[293]. Somewhat less frequently affected are the buccal mucosa, lips, gingiva, and palate. The oral mucosa may present any combination of bullae, infiltrated areas, ecchymoses, and white thickened patches. The picture is from an 8-year-old boy who has a bulla on the alveolar ridge and the particular enamel defect occasionally seen in epidermolysis bullosa.

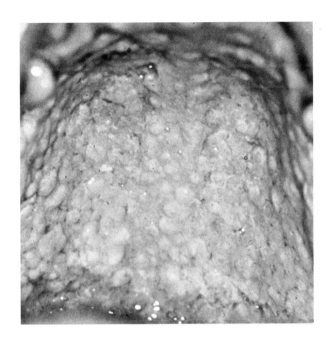

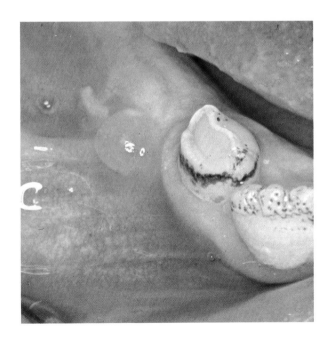

275

Dystrophic epidermolysis bullosa

In patients with the dystrophic type of epidermolysis bullosa, the oral scarring may be so severe that microstomia may result. The buccal and labial sulci may be obliterated by scar tissue, leading to immobility of the lips. The tongue often is bound down to the floor of the mouth, with consequent impairment of tongue mobility and difficulty in deglutition. Squamous cell carcinoma of the involved tongue mucosa has been seen as a complication in older patients. In the skin small epidermal cysts (milia) are frequently found. Such small, well-defined milia may also be observed in the oral mucosa. The illustration shows multiple epi-"dermal" cysts in the palate of a 27-year-old man who suffers from the dystrophic type of epidermolysis bullosa. The same patient was picture in the second edition of this Atlas when he was 14-years old. During the past 13 years the milia have increased in number and size. For the oral mucosa it has been demonstrated[13] that the milia apparently are formed from islands of epithelium detached during the formation of bullae. In the lethal type, the intraoral bullae are remarkably fragile and hemorrhagic[23]. Also in the acquisit type of epidermolysis bullosa oral manifestations have been found[395].

Pseudoxanthoma elasticum

Pseudoxanthoma elasticum (PXE), also known as Grönblad-Strandberg syndrome, is a rare, hereditary disorder of connective tissue, particularly involving the skin, the eyes and the cardiovascular system; also the nervous system may be affected. In most patients the PXE has autosomal recessive inheritance. The disease occurs more frequently in women than in men. The skin lesions appear as cutaneous deposits of yellow material arranged in papules or linear masses most often located to the sides of the neck, and to the axillary, antecubital, inguinal, abdominal and popliteal regions[135]. The cardiovascular involvement expresses itself by early and widespread arterial insufficiency. The oral mucosa may also be the seat of deposits[494]. The illustration opposite shows marked changes of the lower labial mucosa in a 57-year-old woman with PXE. Due to the changes in the underlying connective tissue the mucosa has a yellow color and angioid streaks. A biopsy from this mucosa showed large amounts of thick and twisted collagen fibrils together with calcification inside and around elastic fibers, features which are typical of PXE[136]. Symmetric mucosal changes have been reported on the palate[379].

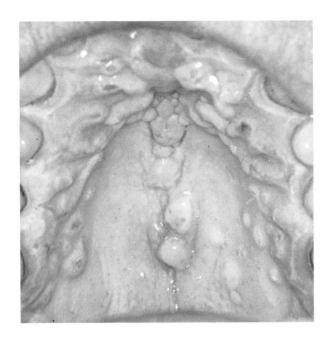

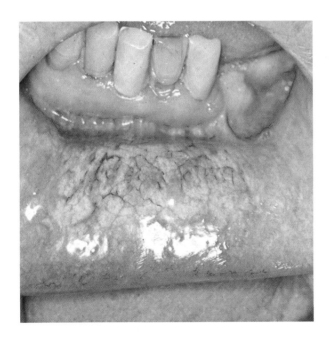

Benign acanthosis nigricans

As mentioned on p. 258, acanthosis nigricans can be divided into several forms. The adult malignant type is dealt with on p. 258. The benign or juvenile type, which is determined by an irregularly dominant gene, is characterized by a hyperpigmentation of the skin, which also becomes furrowed and thickened, with a predilection for the neck, axillae, ano-genital region, and elbow and knee folds. As it is a rare disease and the oral mucosa is seldom examined thoroughly in the course of a general examination, it is difficult to evaluate the frequency of oral manifestations. The tongue and lips are most frequently involved. The papillae on the dorsum of the tongue are hypertrophic and elongated, which gives the tongue a shaggy or prickly appearance. The lips may be markedly enlarged and covered by filiform or papillomatous growths which are especially marked at the commissures of the mouth. When affected, the buccal mucosa presents a diffuse unevenness of its surface with a number of very delicate furrows, as in the 18-year-old girl seen here[420]. It is interesting to compare these changes with those found on the buccal mucosa in the malignant type (p. 258). The latter shows consistently more severe changes than the benign type.

Pachyonychia syndrome

The pachyonychia syndrome, also known as Jadassohn-Lewandowski syndrome, comprises pachyonychia congenita, palmoplantar keratosis and hyperhidrosis, follicular keratosis, and oral leukokeratosis[214]. The syndrome follows an autosomal dominant mode of transmission. In most cases, at birth or soon thereafter, the finger- and toenails become thickened, tubular, and hard, the undersurface being filled with a horny, yellowish-brown material. Palmar and plantar hyperkeratoses are noted in 40 to 65 percent of the cases during the first few years of life. Oral lesions are common in conjunction with pachyonychia. It has been stated that natal teeth and oral leukokeratosis may constitute the earliest clinical manifestation of pachyonychia and that they appear to occur earlier than nail lesions[17]. The dorsum of the tongue is thickened, presenting a white opaque or greyish-white appearance which also involves the margins of the tongue[353] as in the 32-year-old woman shown opposite. Less commonly involved is the buccal mucosa at the interdental line. Clinically, the oral lesions in pachyonychia resemble white sponge nevus and hereditary benign intraepithelial dyskeratosis. (Courtesy of Dr. P. BACH, Aalborg, Denmark).

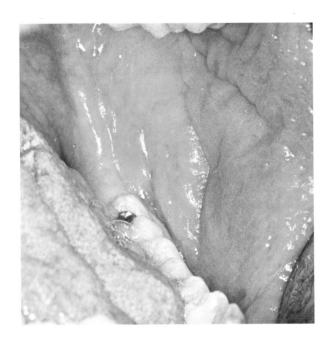

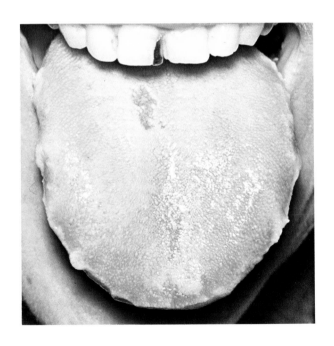

Lingual thyroid

Normally, the thyroid tissue migrates caudally, from an outpouching from the embryonic pharynx, the thyroglossal duct, to the anterolateral surface of the trachea. Occasionally, although not frequently, no thyroid tissue is present in its normal place. Instead it may be located in the base of the tongue, known as lingual thyroid or lingual goiter, either as a complete replacement (65 percent) or in the form of additional thyroid tissue. The heterotopic thyroid tissue also may be found along the normal path of the thyroglossal duct. About 300 cases of lingual thyroid have been reported. The condition appears to occur more frequently among women than among men. A lingual thyroid may be associated with disturbing symptoms such as dysphagia, dysphonia or dyspnea. In one-fifth of the patients there are symptoms of hypothyroidism. A lingual thyroid will present itself as a raised, purplish tumor-like swelling usually about 2 cm to 3 cm in diameter as in the 35-year-old East Indian man seen opposite. The diagnosis of lingual thyroid is now made by the use of scanning with ^{131}I and technetium, which will disclose the exact location of thyroid tissue[451]. (Courtesy of the late Dr. J. ZACHARIAH, Trivandrum, India).

Tuberous sclerosis

Tuberous sclerosis, also known as Bourneville-Pringle syndrome, epiloia, or adenoma sebaceum disseminatum, is a neurocutaneous syndrome characterized by epilepsy, mental deficiency, and adenoma sebaceum[214]. The syndrome is found in about 1 in 300,000 to 500,000 in the general population. Some patients may manifest signs at birth, but in the majority of cases the seizures and skin changes first appear at the age of 2–6 years. Most patients die before they are 20 years old, but some survive into middle age. The facies is the site of numerous adenomata sebacea in the form of small, reddish, flat or rounded, seed-like masses located over the nose, cheeks, nasolabial furrows, and chin. The number seems to increase at puberty. In 11 percent of the cases oral manifestations are present[494] in the form of fibrous growths. Most frequently they are located on the anterior gingiva[498], but they may occur on any oral surface, such as the lip, buccal mucosa, dorsum of the tongue, palate, and uvula. The illustration is of a 41-year-old East Indian with multiple lesions on the buccal mucosa[387]. The lesions usually have the color of the adjacent normal mucosa, but may occasionally be bluish, white, red or yellow. (Courtesy of Drs. R. B. BHONSLE and P. R. MURTI, Ernakulam, India).

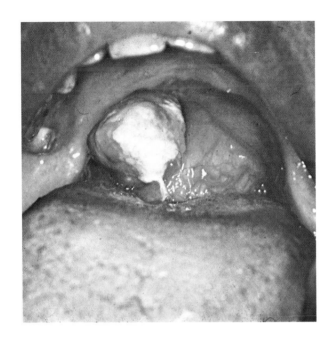

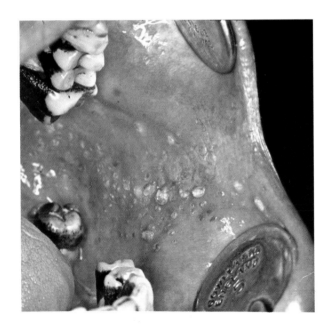

Encephalofacial angiomatosis

Encephalofacial angiomatosis is characterized by a combination of: (1) venous angioma of the leptomeninges overlying the cerebral cortex with ipsilateral angiomatosus lesions of the face and oral mucosa, (2) ipsilateral gyriform calcifications of the brain, (3) epilepsy, and (4) mental retardation. A large number of eponyms have been used in connection with the syndrome, among which the most common is "Sturge-Kalischer-Weber syndrome". The findings in encephalofacial angiomatosis are extremely variable. The anomaly probably arises in exceedingly early stage of embryonic development. On the same side as the cerebral angiomatosis, a nevus flammeus (port-wine nevus) commonly occurs on the face. The facial nevus is present at birth, and in most cases is unilateral, as in the 7-year-old boy seen here, in whom the affected part of the upper lip was hypertrophic. He had suffered from epileptic seizures since birth. The color of the nevus varies from pink to purplish red. A decrease in intensity of color with increasing age has been noted. The nevus is sharply demarcated and usually not markedly elevated. It has been debated whether the distribution of the nevus follows the course of the trigeminal nerve.

Encephalofacial angiomatosis

Oral changes have been described in many of the reported cases of encephalofacial angiomatosis[214]. The most frequent oral sign is involvement of the oral mucosa. Both the buccal and labial mucosa may be the seat of vascular hyperplasia, the color being more bluish red than the normal mucosa. When the lips are affected by the nevus, there is often a macrocheilia[583]. The tongue may be affected, showing either telangiectasia or hemihypertrophy. The gingival mucosa exhibits characteristic changes ranging from slight vascular hyperplasia to monstrous masses making closure of the mouth impossible. The gingival enlargement is soft and purple, and blanches in response to pressure. The color usually stops at the midline of the maxilla, often in contrast to the facial nevus, which stops at the outer margin of the philtrum. Several authors have described an ipsilateral premature eruption of the permanent teeth and, in the same teeth, accelerated tooth formation. The oral changes in the boy pictured above are seen in the picture opposite. The left side of the maxillary oral mucosa was more red than the right side, and there was a more advanced eruption of the maxillary left central incisor and a premature eruption of the lateral incisor.

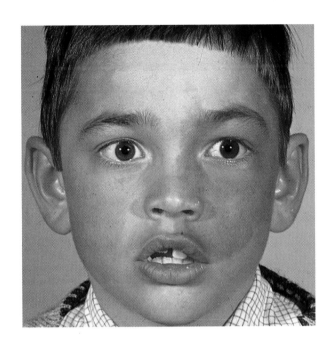

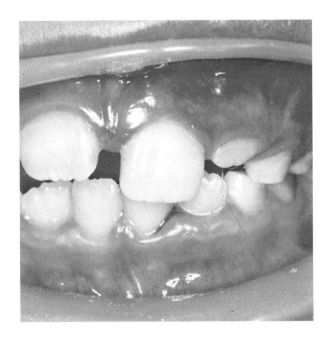

Peutz-Jeghers' syndrome

The syndrome consists of mucocutaneous melanotic pigmentation and intestinal polyposis transmitted as an autosomal dominant disorder with a high degree of penetrance[214]. Polyposis of the gastrointestinal tract is the clinically more important component of the syndrome. The polyps are usually described as benign adenomatous tumors varying in size from 0.5 to 7.0 cm in diameter. Age of onset of symptoms varies from a few weeks to 77 years (average 25 years). In about 50 percent of affected persons, numerous, usually discrete, brown to bluish-black macules are present on the skin, especially about the facial orifices: perioral, perinasal, and periorbital. The skin pigmentation usually appears in infancy and seems to fade somewhat at about puberty. On the vermilion border, especially the lower, and on the oral mucosa, most often on the cheeks, round, oval or irregular, rarely confluent brown macules of variable intensity may be seen. Less frequently pigmented are the palate and gingiva. Only rarely are the tongue and the oral floor involved[303]. The pigmentation is due to an increased amount of melanin in both epithelium and connective tissue. The illustrations is from a 17-year-old man who, since birth, has had pigmentation of skin and oral mucosa. He has been operated on for intestinal polyps.

Acrokeratosis verruciformis

Acrokeratosis verruciformis is an inherited disorder of keratinization. It is inherited as a regular autosomal dominant trait. It was described in 1931 and since a total of 25 cases have appeared in the literature. The onset is usually soon after birth or in early childhood; however, the onset may be delayed until the fifth decade. The clinical manifestations consist of skin-colored, warty papules, flat or convex, present on the knees and elbows, and on the forearms. Small groups or isolated papules may develop in other sites. The verrucous papules may extend to palms and soles[294]. The nails may be thickened and white. Histologically the characteristic feature is hyperkeratosis with a prominent granular cell layer. Oral manifestation may be present as illustrated in the 30-year-old woman opposite. For many years she have been treated for "warts" on arms and legs. The vermilion border is he seat of numerous, small verruciform excrescences. Intraorally, the same lesions are found on the buccal mucosa, the interdental papillae, and the hard palate. A biopsy from the vermilion border shows verruca vulgaris-like changes, whereas biopsies from the buccal mucosa and the gingiva show hyperparakeratosis occasionally with a slight verrucous pattern.

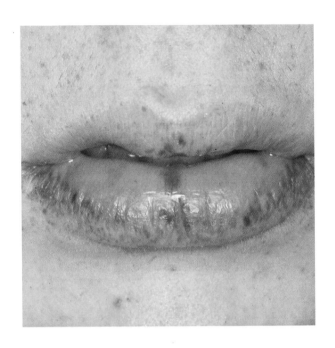

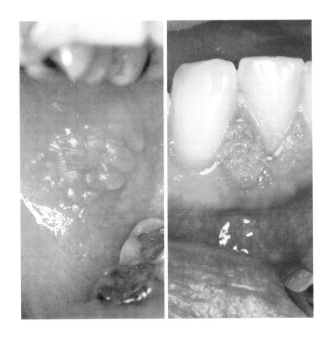

Hereditary mucoepithelial dysplasia

Hereditary mucoepithelial dysplasia is an autosomal, dominantly inherited disorder affecting all of the orificial mucosa with cataracts, follicular keratosis of skin, non-scarring alopecia, bouts of pneumonia, spontaneous pneumothorax, and terminal cor pulmonale[597]. The oral lesion is a fiery red, flat or micropapillary-appearing mucosa most frequently involving the gingiva and hard palate. All oral and pharyngeal mucosa may be involved, however[597]. The patient illustrated is a 9-year-old girl, who had a 4-year younger sister also affected by the disease. The picture shows a fiery red palatal mucosa. The gingiva was also the seat of the same color change which has been present for the last 3 years. Not only the marginal but the entire alveolar gingiva had the same fiery red color giving a strong suspicion of an allergic reaction. The histologic examination of a biopsy from the gingival mucosa revealed in the epithelium corresponding to the rete pegs dyshesive changes with wide intercellular spaces as previously reported[597]. Cytologic examination shows an over-all lack of epithelial maturation. The disease probably represents a defect in the formation and assembly of gap junction and desmosome attachments on the cell surface[597].

SYMPTOMS, SIGNS AND ILL-DEFINED CONDITIONS

Acquired icterus

Icterus or jaundice is the condition recognized clinically by a yellowish discoloration of the plasma, the skin and the mucous membranes caused by staining by bile pigment, bilirubin[478]. The condition often is best detected in the peripheral portions of the ocular conjunctivae. Icterus is frequently the first and sometimes the sole manifestation of liver disease. Disturbances in the mechanisms of uptake, transport, conjugation and biliary excretion of bilirubin are probably responsible for all forms of jaundice. The skin becomes yellow and the deposition of pigment can be observed also in oral mucosa, most often of the hard palate or in the lips when compressed with a glass slide. The illustration opposite is from a 68-year-old man who suffered from an obstruction in the bile duct causing a marked icterus. Not only the skin but also the mucous membrane including the entire oral mucosa were deeply yellow. Depending upon the cause of the icterus, other signs may be pruritus, pain, and enlarged liver. The very light color of the feces gives the best indication whether biliary obstruction is total, intermittent, or decreasing. Characteristic is also the "porter"-stained urine. It should be remembered that the skin may be darker also because of an increased amount of melanin.

286

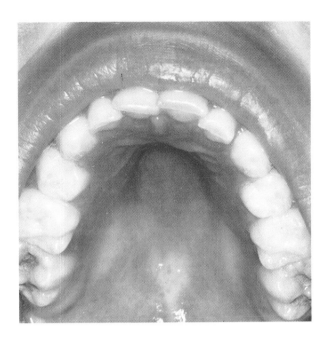

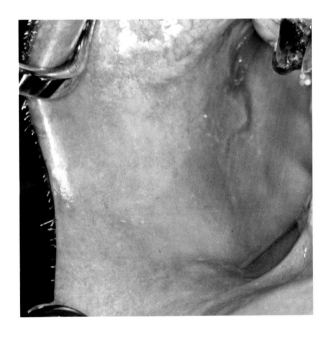

Submucosal ecchymoses after fellatio

Lesions of the oral mucosa due to orogenital contact are reported to be mostly caused by venereal diseases. Physical consequences of oral sexual practice are rarely mentioned, but in 1928 a case was published[46] under the title "*Une affection vénérienne peu banale: le purpura vélo-palatin a vacuo*", which called the attention to palatal ecchymosis as a side effect of fellatio. The illustration opposite is of the palate of a 34-year-old woman who was referred under the diagnosis of a possible oral granuloma annulare. The only complaint was dryness of the throat, which a few days earlier had led to observation of the affection. On the soft palate, a well-demarcated, almost circular lesion was found, about 3 mm broad and with a diameter of 2 cm. The lesion was slightly elevated and consisted of erythema, petechiae and ecchymosis. The lesion and the surrounding mucosa had dilated blood vessels. On direct questioning the patient admitted that she had been practising fellatio the day before the lesion appeared. All signs regressed within a week[603]. It has been suggested that the palatal lesions may be combination of a direct traumatic action with a negative pressure produced at the point of contact at the soft palate[488]. Candidiasis from the penis may be transmitted to the oral mucosa through fellatio[132].

Electric burn

Electric trauma of the mouth may cause very severe lesions, almost worse than those encountered through chemicals or irradiation. Electric burns of the mouth are almost exclusively a phenomenon of childhood in homes where electricity is used carelessly. The problem arises roughly at the age of 4 months when the infants is capable of grasping objects, and it continues as a prominent pattern until approximately the fourth year. When an electric cord and a socket are within reach of an infant, the accident may easily occur. In an instant, the moist lip or the pool of saliva in the labial sulcus creates a short circuit between the cord terminals[434]. An electric area is created, with enough heat to melt steel. Delicate tissues about the lips, alveolar ridge, gingiva, tongue and floor of the mouth are destroyed. This is exemplified in the illustration which is from a 1–2-year-old boy, who got hold of the plug of a vacuum cleaner and put it into his mouth. The typical electric burns of the oral mucosa consist of a painless gray-white coagulated tissue which is demarcated from the contiguous normal-appearing skin by a narrow rim of erythema. The gray zone evolves into brown-black charred tissue and eventually sloughs, leaving an ulcer of varying depth[4].

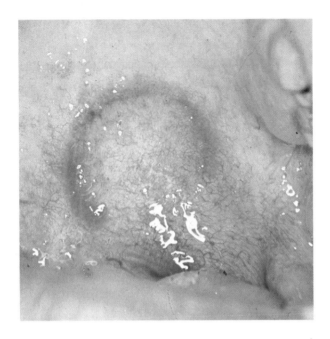

Burn of Internal Organ

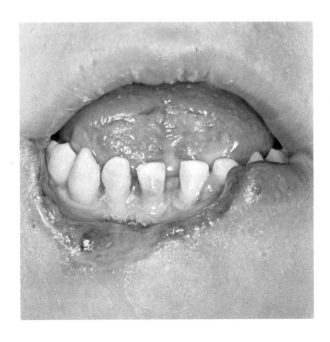

Systemic penicillin administration

Some patients may become hypersensitized to penicillin and, therefore, will develop allergic reactions to the drug. It is estimated that the overall incidence of reactions to penicillin varies from 2 to 8 percent[246]. The rate of fatal anaphylactic reactions after penicillin administration is slightly more than one per milion injections. A patient may become hypersensitive to penicillin by systemic or local administration of the drug, but drinking of milk from cows treated with penicillin may also be a source for eliciting hypersensitivity. Allergic reactions also may develop in patients who have become hypersensitive from a depot of penicillin in a root canal. Apart from anaphylactic shock, the hypersensitivity reactions may comprise a variety of skin eruptions, angioneurotic edema, and oral changes ("stomatitis medicamentosa"). Oral changes occur either during or shortly after systemic treatment with penicillin. The 42-year-old woman seen here developed a vesicular stomatitis on the sixth day after institution of penicillin treatment perorally. Other delayed oral reactions to penicillin treatment are hairy tongue (p. 220) and an atrophic glossitis, most likely an acute atrophic candidiasis. Antibiotics other than penicillin may cause allergic reactions in the oral mucosa.

Quinoline and hydroxyquinoline derivatives

During the Second World War it was found that troops serving more than 6 months in the southwest Pacific developed a pigmentation under the nails and in the hard palate as a result of malarial suppressive therapy with quinacrine (Atebrin). Later reports from Africa and the Pacific areas have confirmed the observation. In a study[95] from New Guinea, the pigmentation was caused by the antimalarial drug amodiaquine (Camoquin). It was found that the pigmentation of the hard palate was of a bluish-gray to almost black color. The palatal pigmentation commenced as irregular patches or streaks of pigment on one or both sides of the midline, eventually coalescing with the increased duration of the suppressive therapy. If the therapy continued for 2 years or more 66 percent of the patients exhibited oral pigmentation, the nature of which was shown to be melanin. The patient seen here is a 68-year-old Danish woman who had received hydroxychloroquine (Ercoquin) for some years for a discoid lupus erythematosus. It is interesting to note that the denture-covered area was devoid of pigment. The permanence of the discoloration is disputed. Some authors describe loss of pigment after end of therapy, whereas others find no loss of pigment[207].

290

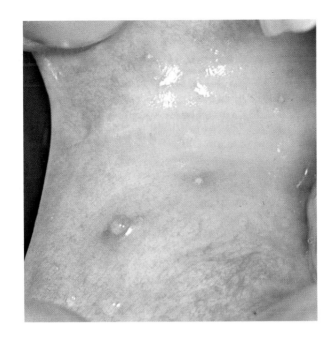

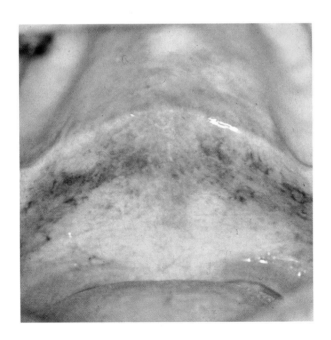

Cytostatic drugs – methotrexate

Since the introduction of cytostatic (cytotoxic) drugs in cancer chemotherapy there have been a number of reports describing several side effects
of the drugs including stomatitis[145]. The patient seen here is a 61-year-
old woman, who has received intraspinal injections of the cytostatic drug
methotrexate for leukemic infiltrates in the central nervous system. After
2 weeks she developed a very painful stomatitis. Lesions similar to the
one seen on the left buccal mucosa were found on the right buccal and
the labial mucosa. The lesions are characterized by erythema, ulcerations
and tags of epithelium seen in many places. The basic aim of cancer
chemotherapy is to maximize the destruction of cancer cells and to minimi-
ze the suppression of normal cells, but, unfortunately, antitumor drugs
cannot distinguish between malignant cells and normal cells and thus are
potentially damaging to both[745]. Clinically, the results of this will be
epithelial atrophy, superficial sloughing, intense reddening, and traumatic
and atraumatic ulceration. From a pilot study[333] it appears that patients
who begin cancer chemotherapy with 5-fluorouracil, adriamycin, and cyclophosphamide with no dental plaque develop less stomatitis than patients with plaque.

Immunosuppressive drugs – azathioprine: stomatitis

Immunosuppressive drugs are used in the treatment of a variety of inflammatory, autoimmune, and other conditions of unknown etiology and are
also used to prevent rejection of organ transplants. The immunosuppressive drugs fall into three groups: antimetabolites such as azathioprine, 6-
mercaptopurine and methotrexate; alkylating agents: cyclophosphamide,
chlorambucil; and antilymphocytic globulins[309]. One of the most widely
used immunosuppressive agents is azathioprine. Its mode of action is
thought to be due to an inhibition of the biosynthesis of purin bases
leading to suppression of nucleic acid and protein synthesis, thereby
inhibiting various immune responses at different stages. The side effects
of the drug are most often seen in rapidly proliferating tissues such as the
bone marrow, the oral mucosa, the gastrointestinal mucosa, and the hair
follicles. An example of oral ulcerations is seen in the illustration, which
is of a 42-year-old man who had a kidney transplantation 10 weeks
before admission to the Dental Department. He has been treated with
azathioprine and after 10 weeks he experienced pain from the gingiva and
the lips. The illustration shows, in several places, small ulcerations, some
of which have a punched-out appearance.

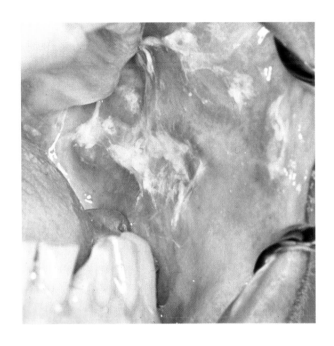

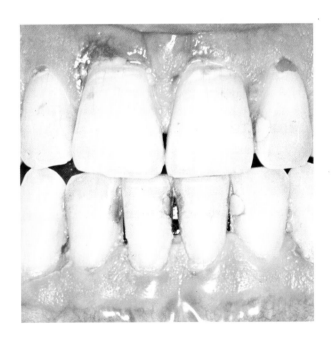

Immunosuppressive drugs – azathioprine: carcinoma

It is a well established fact that renal homograft recipients, treated with immunosuppressive drugs, have an increased incidence of malignant neoplasms between 2–7 percent[40]. It has been suggested that the incidence is approximately 100 times greater than in the general population. The number of patients affected increases with the length of time following transplantation. Thus, an incidence of cancer in renal homograft recipients was found to be 11 percent at 1 year and 24 percent at 5 years[513]. The most frequent malignancy is lymphoma. Development of a Kaposi's sarcoma is illustrated below. With longer periods of follow-up, reports of increased risk for the development of epithelial malignancy, chiefly squamous cell carcinoma have begin to appear. Oral malignancies are rare; so far four carcinomas of tongue and two of floor of mouth have been reported[322, 410]. Carcinoma of the vermilion border have been found in several instances[386]. The picture opposite is of the right buccal mucosa of a 18-year-old man, a non-smoker and a non-drinker, who had a renal homograft 5 years before[423]. A clinical diagnosis of a nodular leukoplakia was followed by a biopsy that revealed a squamous cell carcinoma. The chronic presence of an allograft gives a continual stimulation to the host immune apparatus. This immune stimulation could possibly contribute to the occurrence of malignant tumors[65].

Immunosuppressive drugs – azathioprine: Kaposi's sarcoma

Kaposi's sarcoma er multiple idiopathic hemorrhagic sarcoma is a neoplastic condition, presumably from primitive vasoformative mesenchyme[7], characterized by multiple skin tumors and occasionally visceral involvement. The most frequent occurrence is in the 40–70 year age group. The disease is most common in black persons from Central Africa, but in recent years the disease has been reported as part of AIDS (p. 144) and as a complication to immunosuppressive therapy. Oral lesions may be present with or without concurrent skin lesions. Occasionally oral lesions are the first manifestation of the disease[181]. The oral manifestations, usually well-delineated, raised, soft lesions with a purplish or bluish-red color, are most frequently found in the palate, lips and tongue. Reports[540] have shown the occurrence of Kaposi's sarcoma in patients following renal transplant with concomitant immunosuppressive therapy. The picture demonstrates such a development in a 40-year-old man who had a kidney transplant. He was treated with the immunosuppressive drug azathioprine and developed an herpetic gingivostomatitis[407], which was followed by a Kaposi's sarcoma in four different intraoral locations, of which the gingival lesions is illustrated.

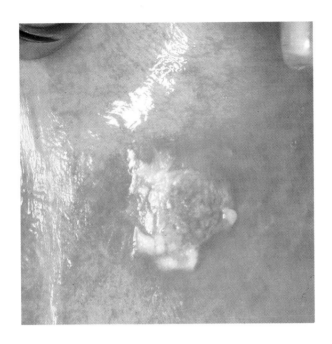

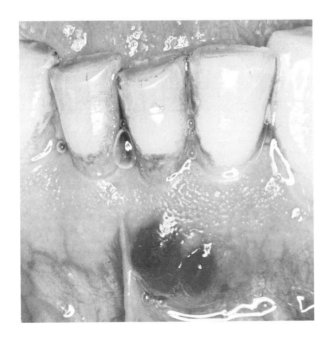

Immunosuppressive drugs – ciclosporin: gingival hyperplasia

Ciclosporin is a powerful immunosuppressive agent discovered in 1972. It is a highly hydrophobic cyclic peptide, obtained from the fermentation broth of two fungi: *Trichoderma polysporum* and *Cylindocarpon lucidum*. It suppresses the antibody responses to T-cell dependent antigens and is now widely used in preventing renal allograft rejection and graft versus host reaction in allogeneic marrow transplantation. Furthermore, ciclosporin is used for several autoimmune disorders. The side effects are less than those caused by the conventional immunosuppressives. The most important side effects are nephro- and hepatotoxicity; less serious are tremor neuropathy, hirsutism and gingival enlargement[449, 614], the latter effect first reported in 1980. The gingival enlargment or hyperplasia appears between 6 to 9 weeks after begin of medication[577]. The favorite site for the hyperplasia is the interdental papillae in the anterior part of both mandible and maxilla. The gingiva in the molar regions may also be affected as seen in the illustration which is from a 59-year-old woman with a bilateral chorioretinitis. After 7 weeks of treatment with ciclosporin she developed marked gingival hyperplasia. When she was taken off the drug, the enlargements became substantially reduced. The presence of plaque and calculus predispose to the development of gingival hyperplasia.

Penicillamine

Since the introduction of penicillamine (dimethylcysteine) in the treatment of scleroderma, heavy metal intoxications, and rheumatoid arthritis, a considerable number of side effects have been reported. One of the less serious complications is a stomatitis. The illustration opposite is of the left buccal mucosa from a 46-year-old woman, who has been treated for a rheumatoid arthritis for 14 years. Three months before admission she began treatment with penicillamine. This led to urticaria and later a stomatitis. Both cheeks are affected by extensive reddening and fibrin-covered ulcerations. Unusual complications of penicillamine treatment are polymyositis – dermatomyositis[413] and pemphigus. Of the latter type several cases have been reported with oral manifestations[241, 313]. These patients had oral lesions, which clinically were similar to ordinary oral pemphigus changes. The diagnosis of pemphigus was made after histologic and immunologic examination. Withdrawal of the penicillamine led to spontaneous resolution of both skin and mucosal ulcerations[241]. Immuno-histochemical findings indicate that the drug eruptions are related to a vasculitis induced by deposition of immune complexes[157].

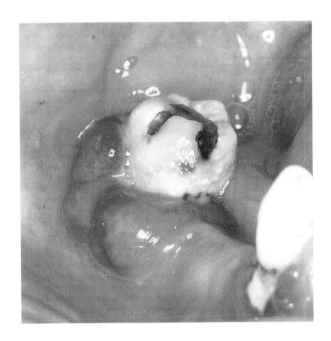

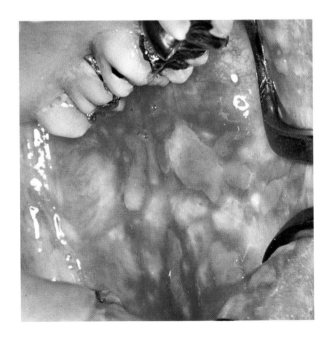

Salicylates

Salicylate intoxication occurs rather frequently, especially in children, and is usually the result of Aspirin (acetylsalicylic acid). Overdosage with salicylates produces the characteristic clinical picture of salicylism comprising nausea, vomiting, sweating, vasodilatation, hyperventilation, tinnitus, deafness and vertigo[438]. Salicylates have important toxic effects on the gastrointestinal tract, the blood and the kidney. Reports on the effect of salicylates upon the oral mucosa have mainly been confined to descriptions of the direct cauterizing effect when the drug is applied in a carious cavity to eliminate pain and the salicylate spreads to the oral mucosa as illustrated on p. 304. Another type of oral reaction is shown in the picture opposite of the lateral border of the tongue in a 30-year-old woman. She suffered from migraine and was taking pills containing acetylsalicylic acid. At first the oral lesions, which appeared on the labial mucosa, floor of mouth, and gingiva, were thought to be of herpetic nature. A provocation test, however, caused an immediate oral reaction upon injection of acetylsalicylic acid. The lesions began as vesicles, which later burst and became fibrin-covered ulcerations as seen in the illustration.

Antirheumatic drugs – indomethacin

Indomethacin is an anti-inflammatory, antipyretic, and analgesic drug that was introduced in 1964 for the treatment of rheumatic and other degenerative joint diseases[226]. Gastrointestinal upsets, headache and vertigo are the commonest side effects of indomethacin[148]. Also a number of allergic reactions, such as skin rashes, angioneurotic edema, and purpuric eruptions have been reported. More rare complications are agranulocytosis, aplastic anemia, and thrombocytopenia. The allergic reactions comprise also oral ulcerations, which have been reported in a number of patients receiving indomethacin. The illustration opposite shows a characteristic oral reaction to the drug. The patient is an 82-year-old woman, who had an inoperable stomach cancer diagnosed 3 months before she was admitted with a painful stomatitis. The clinical examination revealed extensive, fibrin-covered ulcerations on the buccal mucosa; later ulcerations appeared at the labial commissures and bilaterally on the tongue. For 5 years the patient has received indomethacin in the form of Indocid tablets. In a report on oral ulcerations due to indomethacin it has been suggested that the ulcerations develop as a result of an interaction between dentures and the drug[226].

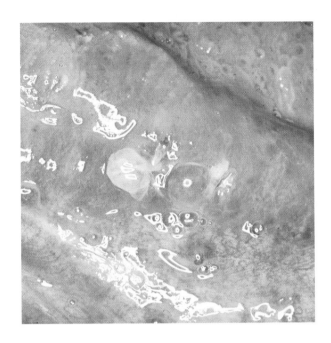

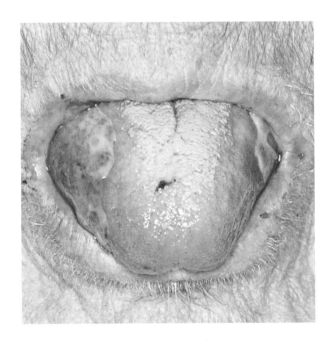

Gold

Gold compounds injected intravenously exert a suppressive effect in rheumatoid arthritis, but they have a potential toxicity. As in the case of other heavy metals, excretion of gold is very slow. Gold is stored in the tissues for a long time and may be detected in traces in the urine for 10 months after administration. The toxic reaction consist in headache, fever, itching, skin eruptions, stomatitis and albuminuria. Of a serious nature are complications such a thrombocytopenia, aplastic anemia, and agranulocytosis. The gold-induced stomatitis may be seen in any part of the oral mucosa, although the inferior surface of the tongue and the floor of the mouth seem to be affected most often. In 18 patients, treated with gold sodium thiosulfate the most frequent mucosal changes were non-specific ulcerations, lichen-like eruptions, atrophy of the filiforme papillae of the tongue and diffuse erythema[209]. A typical lesion is seen in the 65-year-old woman shown here, who had received gold sodium thiosulfate (Sanocrysin) over a period of some weeks. First an itching exanthema appeared on the elbows; then a bilateral ulceration appeared on the palate. Patients receiving gold treatment may develop a contact stomatitis to gold restorations in the mouth[355].

Hydantoin derivatives

No longer ago than 1939, hyperplastic gingival changes were reported in epileptics treated with 5,5-diphenylhydantoin (phenytoin). The use of commercial names for the hyperplasia should be abandoned. The reported incidence of gingival hyperplasia in patients receiving hydantoin derivatives varies from 3 to 62 percent[1]. The incidence of hyperplasia is lower before puberty; there is no sex predilection.[357] The first signs of hyperplasia appear in the interdental papillae, which become enlarged and slightly more red than the adjacent gingiva. The enlarged interdental papillae often will exhibit a stippled surface, as in the illustration from a 27-year-old man who has taken 200 mg phenytoin (Difhydan), daily for 6 years. Later the clinical crowns of the teeth may be completely covered by a solid mass of firmly resilient tissue which does not bleed spontaneously or easily upon probing. Marked pseudopockets may be created by this massive hyperplasia. Hyperplasia is not always associated with clinical symptoms. Phenytoin-induced hyperplasia in edentulous patients is rare. One case has been reported with a massive hyperplasia of the mucosa overlying the unerupted teeth in a 2-year-old boy. The child had had hydantoin medication since birth[472a].

300

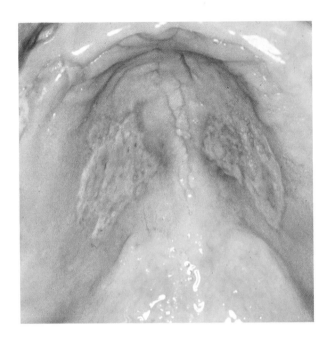

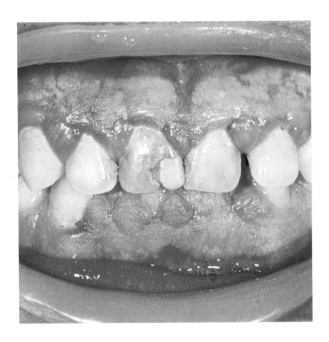

Hydantoin derivatives

The 15-year-old boy seen here had received 300 mg of phenytoin (Difhydan), daily for 2 years. The hyperplasia had here assumed a somewhat monstrous appearance and had involved the attached gingiva. The interdental papilla between the mandibular central incisors was divided into two halves by a delicate groove. This feature, which is observed occasionally in phenytoin gingival hyperplasia, is due to an epithelial rete ridge growing down and separating the hyperplastic collagenous tissue into two halves. Quite often the clinical picture becomes modified by inflammatory changes whereby the gingiva assumes a fiery red color, and a purulent discharge may appear from the pockets. A positive correlation has been demonstrated between the overgrowth severity and gingival inflammation, probing depths, calculus accumulation, plaque score and the measurement gingival margin to mucogingival junction. In the same study no correlation was observed between lesion severity and patient age, daily drug usage, plasma or saliva phenytoin level, or salivary concentration of the major phenytoin metabolite[238]. The mechanism behind the gingival hyperplasia is still unknown. A new finding is a significant increase in the non-collagenous matrix, and a decrease in the collagenous matrix[131].

Paraformaldehyde

Chemical injuries of a chronic nature may be caused by prolonged use of certain drugs by the patient or by incorrect use of caustics by the dentist, causing a contact necrosis. To the first group belongs the harmful influence of regular mouthwash with concentrated sodium perborate. Other agents known to produce oral mucosa changes by misuse are iodine, phenol, and silver nitrate. In some countries paraformaldehyde is used, or has been used, for pulp mummification, often with amydricaine chloride added as an anesthetic. Paraform, which is prepared by polymerizing formic aldehyde by heat, liberates formaldehyde vapors at ordinary temperature. It is a caustic, and may cause undesirable side effects if not properly safeguarded. The illustration shows a necrotic vestibular interdental papilla between the first and second molars. The patient, a 24-year-old man, had a chronic pulpitis in the first molar. The dentist applied paraformaldehyde to devitalize the pulp, but was not cautious enough when sealing the cavity with zinc oxide-eugenol. Before the cement set, some paraform was squeezed out into the interdental space, causing necrosis of the interdental papillae and of the osseous septum.

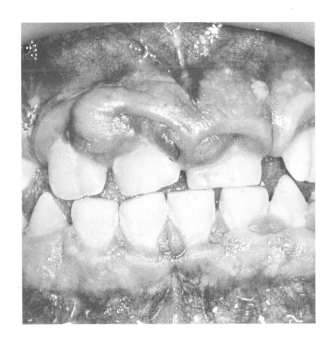

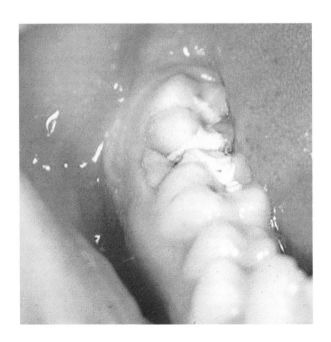

Chlorhexidine

Chlorhexidine is an antibacterial agent with activity against Gram-positive and Gram-negative bacteria as well as yeasts. The toxicity of chlorhexidine is low. Chlorhexidine in concentrations of 0.2 and 0.1 percent has been shown to be efficient in the prevention of induced plaque formation and gingivitis in man[346]. Side effects such as discolorations of teeth and tongue and interference with taste have been observed not too infrequently. More rare is desquamation of the oral epithelium which was found in 10 persons among 148 men rinsing with either 0.2 or 0.1 percent chlorhexidine daily for 17 weeks[194]. In seven instances the lesions were small and lasted only for a short period. However, in three patients the lesions were more severe as in the 18-year-old man illustrated opposite. The patient had been rinsing his mouth with 0.2 percent chlorhexidine gluconate. He then developed a burning sensation of the oral mucosa and pain associated with erythema of the gingiva and buccal groove. In some areas white desquamations of the epithelium appeared. Upon scraping small erosions were seen[481]. The lesions disappeared when the concentration of chlorhexidine was reduced to 0.1 percent.

Acetylsalicylic acid (Aspirin burn)

A chemical burn frequently observed in the mouth is caused by placing tablets containing acetylsalicylic acid in the vestibular sulcus close to a tooth which gives pain. As the original trade name for acetylsalicylic acid is Aspirin, the ensuing lesion is often called an Aspirin burn. It appears shortly after the tablet has been placed in position. A burning sensation of the mucosa is experienced and the affected area becomes blanched or white. Short exposures of the drug to the mucosa cause a white and wrinkled lesion, while longer exposures lead to soggy, white, and swollen lesions[610]. The illustration is of a 31-year-old man who tried to alleviate severe pain in his maxillary right first premolar by placing a tablet of acetylsalicylic acid in the vestibular sulcus. The lesion, which was quite extensive, belongs to the group of soggy and swollen lesions. Oral Aspirin burn is the result of mucosal slough due to coagulation of the protein in the superficial epithelial cells[389] caused by acetylsalicylic acid's pH of 3.5. Oral chemical burns may also be caused by careless handling of various medications, such as cavity varnish or hydrofluoric acid. Excess consumption of fresh fruit and fresh juices may cause a chemical burn of the masticatory mucosa in association with abusive oral hygiene practices[563].

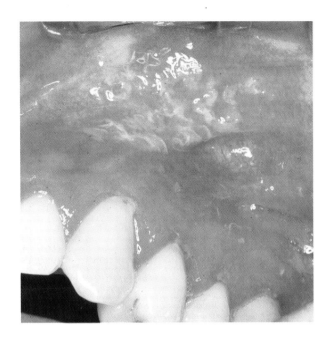

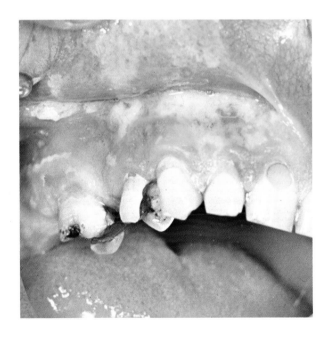

Lead

Lead intoxication is still one of the most important industrial hazards. Gingival pigmentation caused by lead has also been observed in patients with a history of pica sometimes in mentally retarded[336]. The intoxication is characterized by a generalized muscular discomfort, headache, loss of weight, constipation, lead colic, anemia, a grayish color of the skin, and gingival discoloration. The gingival lead line ("halo saturninus", "Burton's line") may be the sign which leads to recognition of the lead intoxication. The lead line is bluish-black, a few millimeters in width, and follows the marginal gingiva. It is caused by the deposition of isoluble lead sulfide in the capillary endothelial cells and in histiocytes. The lead line is not seen in edentulous persons[370], and in patients with a dark skin it may be difficult to distinguish from a physiologic gingival pigmentation[212]. The differential diagnosis from calculus can be made by placing a small strip of paper in the gingival pocket, as illustrated in the picture, where the lead line is clearly seen separated from the tooth. The insert shows the excised gingival tissue, demonstrating the deposit of lead inside the pocket. The patient was a 47-year-old man who had been working for 6 months as a metal grinder.

Mercury

Intoxication by mercury may be due either to the use of mercury-containing drugs, primarily in the form of diuretics, or as an industrial hazard. The symptoms of a systemic mercury intoxication include general malaise, nausea, anorexia, bloody diarrhea, and oliguria. The intoxication causes cardiac arrest, hemorrhagic colitis, renal damage, and oral changes. The oral manifestations comprise excessive salivation, metallic taste, discoloration of the mucous membrane, and stomatitis. The discoloration is rarely seen. The gingiva becomes red, swollen, and necrotic; in late stages the teeth are loose and the alveolar bone may become exposed and necrotic. The oral mucosal lesions consist of grayish-yellow membranes, often with a circinate appearance. The affected areas may be quite extensive and necrotic[444]. The patient seen here is a 48-year-old man who had been working in direct contact with mercury in a plant. After 1 week he suffered a general malaise, sore throat, and bleeding gingiva. Besides the affections on the marginal and attached gingiva he had similar lesions on the buccal mucosa and border of the tongue. The urine contained 11,000 γ/l mercury[318]. The normal value is 10 γ/l.

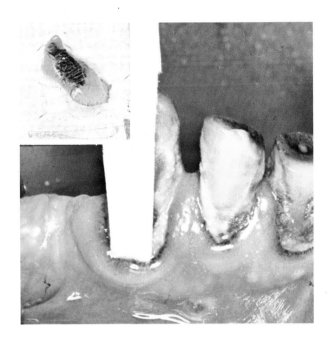

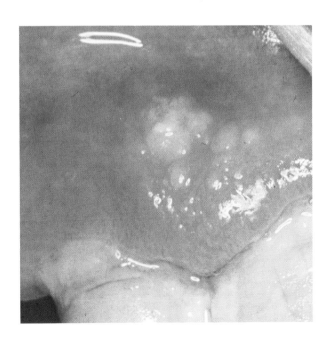

307

Radiation mucositis

The use of roentgentherapy and curietherapy in the treatment of oral malignant diseases may have deleterious effects on adjacent normal oral structures. Best known is osteoradionecrosis, which is still a rather frequent complication. Another adverse effect is the radiation mucositis of the oral mucosa. The first changes occur toward the end of the first week of therapy and consist of a reddening of the buccal mucosa. By the middle of the second week, white patches appear on the labial and buccal mucosa and tongue[465]. With continued treatment the mucositis becomes more severe, the tongue becomes the site of a glossitis, and ulcerations may occur. If salivary glands have been in the radiation field, the patients may subsequently experience a loss of taste, and sometimes mouth bitterness and a dryness of the mouth. The degree of these signs and symptoms is dose-related and there is a gradual improvement once radiation has ceased[10]. The patient seen here is a 46-year-old woman who has received radium mould and cobalt radiation on a carcinoma in the floor of the mouth. The lips, the inferior surface of the tongue, and the floor of the mouth are the site of an extensive mucositis characterized by fibrin-covered ulcerations and marked erythema.

Angioneurotic edema

The illustration shows a swelling of tongue, especially of the right side, in a 43-year-old man[392]. For 2 years the patient has suffered from recurrent, sometimes daily, attacks of urticaria on the skin and swelling of lips and tongue. Laboratory studies, including a number of patch tests, did not reveal anything abnormal. A radiographic examination of the teeth disclosed three teeth with periapical osteitis. These foci were eliminated but it did not improve either the urticaria or the edema. As there was no hereditary background, the condition was diagnosed as a non-hereditary angioneurotic edema. There are two types of angioneurotic edema, a non-hereditary type and a hereditary type. Both types have the same cutaneous symptoms, but the hereditary type has often visceral manifestations. The non-hereditary type is rather easy to diagnose, as the lesion is highly distinctive. The absence of pain, heat and redness differentiates this condition from an acute infective process[115]. The lesion in angioneurotic edema is usually single, but there can be multiple lesions occasionally. In some cases the edema gradually develops over a number of hours, whereas other cases acquire a swelling, which appears with astonishing suddenness[115].

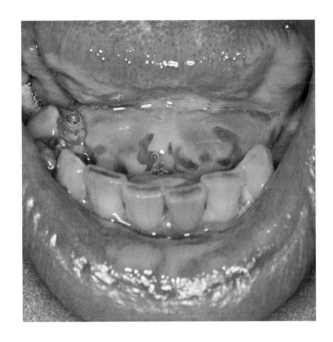

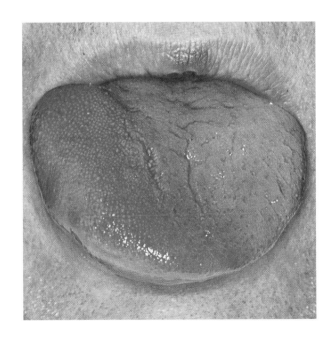

Amalgam tattoo

Pigmentation of the oral mucosa caused by amalgam (a mixture of silver, tin and mercury,) the so-called amalgam tattoo, is a well-known lesion. In an unselected Swedish population sample an oral amalgan tattoo was found in 8 percent[24]. In most cases it is the gingiva and alveolar mucosa which become the site of the discoloration[84]. Clinically, the amalgam tattoo presents itself as a well-defined pigmented area with a bluish, blackish or slate grey color. It is characteristic that the pigmented spot is not elevated. The illustration shows a typical example of amalgam tattoo located on the attached gingiva in a 25-year-old man. The amalgam may reach the mucosa in different ways. It may occur as a result of fracture of a silver amalgam filling during tooth extraction and inclusion of the amalgam fragments in the extraction wound; when the wound heals the amalgam will lie near the surface of the mucosa. Another cause of amalgam tattoo is when small particles of amalgam are spilled into the periodontal tissues during the filling procedure of an approximal cavity. Amalgam may also become displaced during surgical endodontic procedures where the apices are sealed with amalgam[538]. The histologic aspects of amalgam tattoo are described in the text below.

Metal tattoo

It is part of the experience of all dentists that a bur or a disk during dental operative procedures may slip and injure the oral mucosa. In most such cases the healing is fast and uneventful. Occasionally, however, a permanent mark may be left in the form of a pigmented area. This is caused by the presence of particles of metal. The illustration opposite shows a discoloration of the left buccal mucosa in a 56-year-old man who was exposed to an accident some years before the present examination. The patient's dentist used a carborundum disk which slipped and pierced into the buccal mucosa. Particles of ebonite remained in the area and have caused the pigmented spot. In pigmented spots caused by amalgam, the metal particles occur both in fragments associated with a foreign body reaction and in a finely dispersed form along the fibers of the connective tissue causing an *in vivo* silver stain of the precollagenous fibers. A metal tattoo also may be seen in cases where the root canal of a primary tooth has been filled with a silver-containing material. When the root and bone are resorbed, the metal may be visible through the mucosa[404]. The most important differential diagnosis for all pigmented areas is the melanoma which, in contrast to the flat metallic deposits, is an elevated lesion.

310

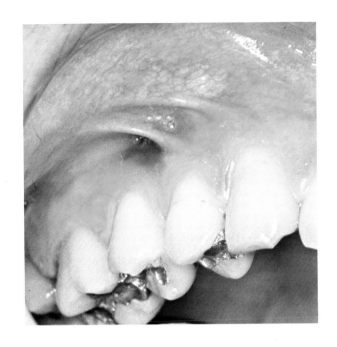

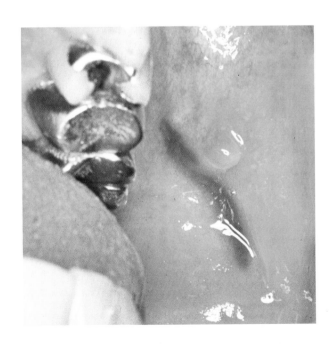

Cotton roll "stomatitis"

It is the experience of most dentists that cotton rolls placed in the vestibular sulcus sometimes may give rise to an injury of the mucosa. In the majority of cases the lesion is found on the maxillary gingiva. When the cotton roll in such cases is removed, the superficial layers of the roll adhere to the underlying mucosa, and within a day or two a fibrin-covered lesion develops. The lesion, which is superficial and shows a fast spontaneous healing, may be quite painful. The illustration is from a 24-year-old woman who developed a cotton roll "stomatitis" after a roll had been placed in the sulcus. The etiology of the cotton roll "stomatitis" is not completely understood. A rough removal of the roll combined with a drying of the mucosa by the roll may be contributory factors; in the area most often affected, very small amounts of saliva are present as the patient leans his head backwards in the dental chair. It has also been suggested that the rolls may contain irritating substances or that the lesion is caused by an allergic reaction, but these possbilities are very remote[169]. Also a local ischemia caused by an anesthetic should be considered as an etiologic factor.

Vaccinia of oral mucosa

If a child vaccinated against smallpox and, with the fingers, transfers the vaccine to other parts of the body, a localized secondary inoculation may occur. In order to accept a case as vaccinia, the lesion on the site of the secondary inoculation shall be consistent with the proliferation and necrosis which characterize the primary vaccinia[497]. The oral mucosa may become the site of a secondary inoculation as in the 8-year-old mentally retarded girl shown opposite. The child was vaccinated, against smallpox, in the shoulder. Ten days later, whitish, centrally umbilicated lesions appeared on the left commissure and on the tongue because the child had had her fingers on the vaccination site and carried the vaccine into her mouth. There were six lesions on the dorsum of the tongue. The vaccinia lesions on the oral mucosa have a tendency to coalesce and produce a plaque with a serpiginous outline and elevated margins[586]. The oral lesions have been divided into three categories: pustular, papular and diphtheric[405]. The tongue is the most frequently involved site in the oral cavity with the lips (commissures), gingiva, buccal mucosa, tonsils, and uvula involved less frequently. (Courtesy of Dr. B. RUSSELL, Copenhagen, Denmark).

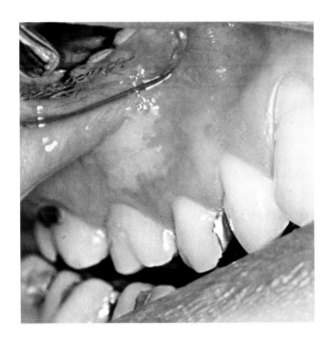

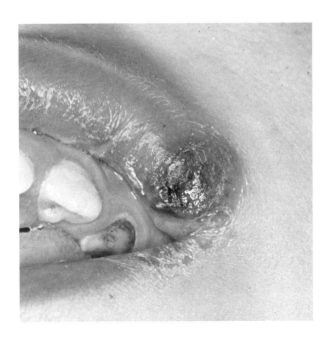

Graft-versus-host reaction

The graft-versus-host reaction (GVHR) or graft-versus-host disease is a complex, multisystem immunologic phenomenon characterized by the engraftment of immunocompetent cells from one individual to a host who is not only immunodeficient, but who possesses transplantation isoantigens foreign to the graft and therefore capable of stimulating it[63]. The reported incidence of GVHR following bone marrow transplantation from various centers ranges from 20 to 50 percent. The acute form of GVHR is characterized by a skin rash, hepatitis, and diarrhea, with the skin manifestations as the most important aspect of GVHR. Oral manifestations may appear 21 to 43 days after the transplantation as fine papules, lichenoid and/or desquamative reactions[44]. A chronic form may follow the acute form or arise *de novo* about 100 days after the transplantation. A constant feature of chronic GVHR is a lichen planus-like skin eruption progressing to scleroderma. Oral manifestations may appear in the form of a lichenoid keratosis and ulcerations. The latter change is a marked feature in the 18-year-old man illustrated opposite. He suffered from acute lymphatic leukemia and had a bone marrow transplantation performed. After 7 weeks lichenoid changes appeared in several areas of the oral mucosa. Later extensive ulcerations developed.

Graft-versus-host reaction

The histologic changes characterizing the GVHR have separated into two distinct processes (1) a lymphoid response and (2) aggressor lymphocyte reaction (destructive epithelial lesions[524]). Target areas for destructive epithelial lesions include epithelia of skin, squamous mucous membranes, liver, and small and large intestines. The oral epithelium will show focal coagulation necrosis. The necrotic cells may drop down into lamin propria as "nummified" bodies[524]. Such changes may easily explain the drastic features observed clinically as in the 43-year-old woman illustrated. Five months before the picture was taken, the patient had a bone marrow transplantation performed because of an aplastic anemia. The oral manifestations may be the first sign of a GVHR. Recent investigators[273] have analyzed labial minor gland salivary flow rate and sodium concentration in patients with GVHR. The labial saliva sodium concentration were elevated and the increase associated with inflammation and destruction of minor salivary gland acini and ducts. Thus, if a bone marrow transplant recipient is found to have an elevated labial saliva sodium level, then the probability that he has pathologic labial gland changes is 91 present.

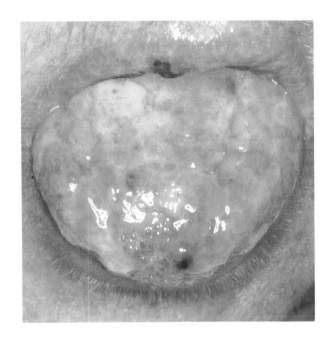

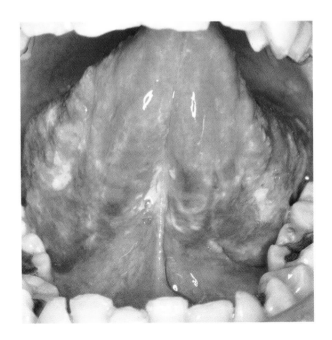

Bibliography

1. Aas E. Hyperplasia gingivae diphenyl-hydantoinea. A clinical, histological, and biochemical study. *Acta Odontol Scand* 1963: **21**: Suppl. 34.
2. Abrams AM, Finch FM. Sialoadenoma papilliferum. A previously unreported salivary gland tumor. *Cancer* 1969; **24**: 1057–63.
3. Abrahams AM, Melrose RJ, Howell FV. Necrotizing sialometaplasia: a disease simulating malignancy. *Cancer* 1973; **32**: 130–5.
4. Ackerman A, Goldfaden GL. Electrical burns of the mouth in children. *Arch Dermatol* 1971; **104**: 309–11.
5. Adams D, Carney JS, Dicks DA. Pregnancy gingivitis: a survey of 100 antenatal patients. *J Dent* 1974; **2**: 106–10.
6. Adatia AK. Significance of jaw lesions in Burkitt's lymphoma. *Br Dent J* 1978; **145**: 263–6.
7. Akhtar M, Bunnuan H, Ali MA, Godwin JT. Kaposi's sarcoma in renal transplant recipients. *Cancer* 1984; **53**: 258–66.
8. Akker HP van der, Bays RA, Becker AE. Plunging or cervical ranula: review of the literature and report of 4 cases. *J Max-Fac Surg* 1978; **6**: 286–93.
9. Allan D, Straton AG. Chronic granulomatous disease with associated oral lesions. *Br Dent J* 1983; **154**: 110–2.
10. Al-Tikriti U, Martin MV, Bramley PA. A pilot study of the clinical effects of irradiation on the oral tissues. *Br J Oral Max-Fac Surg* 1984; **22**: 77–86.
11. Andersen H, Holst G. Dental changes in some endocrine disorders. *Acta Paediatr* (Uppsala) 1959; Suppl. 118: 157.
12. Anderson DL. Cause and prevention of lip cancer *J Can Dent Assoc* 1971; **37**: 138–42.
13. Andreasen JO, Hjørting-Hansen E, Ulmansky M, Pindborg JJ. Milia formation in oral lesions in epidermolysis bullosa. *Acta Pathol Microbiol Scand* 1965; **63**: 37–41.
14. Andreasen JO, Pindborg JJ. Cancerudvikling i oral lichen planus. *Nord Med* 1963; **70**: 861–6.
15. Angelopoulos AP. Pyogenic granuloma of the oral cavity: statistical analysis of its clinical features. *J Oral Surg* 1971; **29**: 840–7.
16. Anneroth G, Heimdahl A. Syndrome of multiple mucosal neurofibromas, pheochromocytoma and medullary thyroid carcinoma. Report of a case. *Int J Oral Surg* 1978; **7**: 126–31.
17. Anneroth G, Isacsson G, Lagerholm B, Lindvall A-M, Thyresson N. Pachyonychia congenita. A clinical, histological and microradiographic study with special reference to oral manifestations. *Acta Dermatovenerol* 1975; **55**: 387–94.
18. Araki S, Murata K, Ushio K, Sakai R. Dose-response relationship between tobacco consumption and melanin pigmentation in the attached gingiva. *Arch Environ Health* 1983; **38**: 375–8.
19. Archard HO, Heck JW, Stanley HR. Focal epithelial hyperplasia: an unusual oral mucosal lesion found in Indian children. *Oral Surg* 1965; **20**: 201–12.
20. Arendorf TM, Walker DM. Tobacco and denture wearing as local aetiological factors in median rhomboid glossitis. *Int J Oral Surg* 1984; **13**: 411–5.
21. Arendorft TM, Walker DM, Kingdom RJ, Roll JRS, Newcombe RG. Tobacco smoking and denture wearing in oral candidal leukoplakia. *Br Dent J* 1983; **155**: 340–3.
22. Aronson K, Soltani K. Chronic mucocutaneous candidosis: a review. *Mycopathologia* 1976; **60**: 17–25.
23. Arwill T, Bergenholtz A, Thilander H. Epidermolysis bullosa hereditaria. V. The ultrastructure of oral mucosa and skin in four cases of the letalis form. *Acta Pathol Microbiol Scand* 1968; **74**: 311–24.
24. Axéll T. *A prevalence study of oral mucosal lesions in an adult Swedish population.* Thesis. *Odontol Revy* 1976; **27**. Suppl. 36.
25. Axéll T, Hedin A. Epidemiologic study of excessive oral melanin pigmentation with

special reference to the influence of tobacco habits. *Scand J Dent Res* 1982; **90**: 434–42.

26. AXÉLL T, HENRICSSON V. Leukoedema – an epidemiologic study with special reference to the influence of tobacco habits. *Community Dent Oral Epidemiol* 1981; **9**: 142–6.

27. AXÉLL T, HENRICSSON V. Association between recurrent aphthous ulcers and tobacco habits. *Scand J Dent Res* 1985; **95**: in press.

28. AXÉLL T, HOLMSTRUP P, KRAMER IRH, PINDBORG JJ, SHEAR M. International seminar on oral leukoplakia and associated lesions related to tobacco habits. *Community Dent Oral Epidemiol* 1984; **12**: 145–54.

29. AXÉLL T, KOCH G. Traumatic ulcerative gingival lesion. *J Clin Periodontol* 1982; **9**: 178–83.

30. AXELSEN NH. Human precipitins against a microorganism (Candida albicans) demonstrated by means of quantitative immunoelectrophoresis. *Clin Exp Immunol* 1971; **9**: 749–52.

31. AZAZ B, LUSTMAN J. Keratoacanthoma of the lower lip. Review of the literature and report of a case. *Oral Surg* 1974; **38**: 918–27.

32. BADEN E, JONES JR, KHEDEKAR R, BURNS WA. Neurofibromatosis of the tongue: a light and electronmicroscopic study with review of the literature from 1849 to 1981. *J Oral Med* 1984; **39**: 157–64.

33. BADGER GR. Oral signs of chickenpox (varicella): report of two cases. *J Dent Child* 1980; **47**: 349–51.

34. BACHNI PC, PAYOT P, TSAI C-C, CIMASONI G. Periodontal status associated with chronic neutropenia. *J Clin Periodontol* 1983; **10**: 222–30.

35. BAKER AB, ed. *Clinical neurology*. Vol. 3. New York: Paul B Hoeber, 1955.

36. BANG G. Acanthosis nigricans maligna: paraneoplasia with oral manifestations. *Oral Surg* 1970; **29**: 370–5.

37. BÁNÓCZY J, ROED-PETERSEN B, PINDBORG JJ, INOVAY J. Clinical and histologic studies on electrogalvanically induced oral white lesions. *Oral Surg* 1979; **48**: 319–23.

38. BÁNÓCZY J, SUGÁR L, FRITHIOF L. White sponge nevus: leukoedema exfoliativum mucosae oris. A report on forty-five cases. *Swed Dent J* 1973; **66**: 481–93.

39. BÁNÓCZY J, SZABÓ L, CSIBA A. Migratory glossitis. A clinical-histologic review of seventy cases. *Oral Surg* 1975; **39**: 113–21.

40. BARA J. Les manifestations bucco-maxillo-faciales de la syphilis tertiaire. *Actualités Odonto-Stomatol* 1951; No. 13: 7–43.

41. BARKER DS, LUCAS RB. Localised fibrous overgrowths of the oral mucosa. *Br J Oral Surg* 1967; **5**: 86–92.

42. BARKIN ME, BOYD JP, COHEN S. Acute allergic reaction to eugenol. *Oral Surg* 1984; **57**: 441–2.

43. BARRETT AP. Gingival lesions in leukemia: a classification. *J Periodontol* 1984; **55**: 585–8.

44. BARRETT AP, BILOUS M. Oral patterns of acute and chronic graft-v-host disease. *Arch Dermatol* 1984; **120**: 1461–5.

45. BARRETT AP, TVEVSKY J, GRIFFITHS CJ. Thrombocytopenia induced by quinine. *Oral Surg* 1983; **55**: 351–4.

46. BARTHÉLEMEY R. Une affection vénérienne peu banale: le purpura vélo-palatin "a vacuo". *Ann Malad Vénér* 1928; **23**: 451–3.

47. BASKER RM, STURDEE DW, DAVENPORT JC. Patients with burning mouth: a clinical investigation of causative factors, including the climacteric and diabetes. *Br Dent J* 1978; **145**: 9–16.

48. BASU MK, ASQUITH P, THOMPSON RA, COOKE WT. Oral manifestations of Crohn's disease. *Gut* 1975; **16**: 249–54.

49. BATHARD-SMITH PJ, COONAR HS, MARKUS AF. Hodgkin's disease presenting intra-orally. *Br J Oral Surg* 1978–79; **16**: 64–9.

50. BATSAKIS JG, BRANNON RB, SCIUBBA JJ. Monomorphic adenomas of major salivary glands: a histologic study of 96 tumors. *Clin Otolaryngol* 1981; **6**: 129–43.

51. BAUGHMAN RA. Median rhomboid glossitis: a developmental anomaly? *Oral Surg* 1971; **31**: 56–65.

318

52. BECKER J, LÖNING T, REICHART P, HARTMANN N. Oral lichen planus: characterization of immmunocompetent cells with hybridoma antibodies. *J Oral Pathol* 1983; **12**: 117–23.
53. BENNETT DE. Histoplasmosis of the oral cavity and larynx. A clinicopathologic study. *Arch Intern Med* 1967; **120**: 417–27.
54. BERGENDAL T, ISACSSON G. A combined clinical mycological and histological study of denture stomatitis. *Acta Odontol Scand* 1983; **41**: 33–44.
55. BERGENHOLTZ A, HOFER P-Å, ÖHMAN J. Oral, pharyngeal and laryngeal manifestations in Urbach-Wiethe disease. *Ann Clin Res* 1977; **9**: 1–7.
56. BERNIER JL, CLARK ML. Squamous cell carcinoma of the lip. A critical statistical and morphological analysis of 835 cases. *Milit Surg* 1951; **109**: 379–405.
57. BERNSTEIN ML, McDONALD JS. Oral lesions in Crohn's disease: report of two cases and update of the literature. *Oral Surg* 1978; **46**: 234–45.
58. BERRY HH, LANDWERLEN JR. Cigarette smoker's lip lesion in psychiatric patients. *J Am Dent Assoc* 1973; **86**: 657–62.
59. BERTRAM U. *Xerostomia. Clinical aspects, pathology and pathogenesis.* Thesis. *Acta Odontol Scand* 1967; **25**: Suppl. 49.
60. BETHMANN W. Lappenfibrosen. *Dtsch Stomatol* 1962; **2**: 83–8.
61. BEVERIDGE BR, BANNERMAN RM, EVANSON JM, WITTS LJ. Hypochromic anaemia. A retrospective study and follow-up of 378 inpatients. *Q J Med* 1965; **34**: 145–61.
62. BHASKAR SN, JACOWAY JR. Pyogenic granuloma – clinical features, incidence, histology and result of treatment: report of 242 cases. *J Oral Surg* 1966; **24**: 391–8.
63. BILLINGHAM RE. The biology of graft-versus-host reactions. *Harv Lect Ser* 1966; **62**: 21–78.
64. BINNIE WH, DAY RCB, LYNN AH. Lymphosarcoma presenting with oral symptoms. *Br Dent J* 1971; **130**: 235–8.
65. BIRKELAND SA. Malignant tumors in renal transplant patients. *Cancer* 1983; **51**: 1571–5.
66. BLAKE GC. Acute streptococcal gingivitis. *Dent Practit Dent Rec* 1959; **10**: 43–5.
67. BLANK H, RAKE G. *Viral and rickettsial diseases of the skin, eye and mucous membranes of man.* London: JA Churchill Ltd, 1955.
68. BLANTON PL, HURT WC, LARGEUT MD. Oral factitious injuries. *J Periodontol* 1977; **48**: 33–7.
69. BLASBERG B, JORDAN-KNOX A, CONKLIN RJ. Gingival ulceration due to improper toothbrushing. *J Can Dent Assoc* 1981; **47**: 462–4.
70. BLOK P, DELDEN L VAN, WAAL I VAN DER. Non-Hodgkin's lymphoma of the hard palate. *Oral Surg* 1979; **47**: 445–52.
71. BORELLO E, POEX A. Blastomycose sud-américaine. *Rev Stomatol* (Paris) 1970; **71**: 495–9.
72. BRANDRUP F, KOCH C, PETRI M, SCHIØDT M, JOHANSEN KS. Discoid lupus erythematosus-like lesions and stomatitis in female carriers of X-linked chronic granulomatous disease. *Br J Dermatol* 1981; **104**: 495–500.
73. BRAUDE AI. Other deep mycoses. In: WINTROBE MM *et al. Harrison's principles of internal medicine.* New York: McGraw-Hill Book Company, 1974; 906–9.
74. BROCHERIOU C, CREPY C, GUILBERT F, LARTIGAU G, PAYEN J, RECOING J. Tumeurs des glandes salivaires accessoires de la cavité buccale. *Bull Cancer* (Paris) 1980; **67**: 29–37.
75. BROCHERIOU C, SZPIRGLAS H, DE ROQUANCOURT A, BERTRAND JC. Mélanome malin developpé sur mélanose circonscrite précancereuse intra-buccale (mélanose de Dubreuilh): étude de deux cas. *Acta Stomatol Belg* 1980; **77**: 115–28.
76. BROCKBANK J. Hemangiopericytoma of the oral cavity: report of case and review of literature. *J Oral Surg* 1979; **37**: 659–64.
77. BROGAN WF, MURPHY BP. The effects of zero population growth on the incidence of cleft lip and palate in Western Australia. *Med J Aust* 1978; **1**: 126–30.
78. BRO-JØRGENSEN A, JENSEN T. Gonococcal tonsillar infections. *Br Med J* 1971; **4**: 660–1.
79. BROOK IM, KING DJ, MILLER ID. Chronic granulomatous cheilitis and its relationship to Crohn's disease. *Oral Surg* 1983; **56**: 405–7.
80. BROOKE RI. Exfoliative cheilitis. *Oral Surg* 1978; **45**: 52–5.

319

81. BROOKE RI, SAPP JP. Herpetiform ulceration. *Oral Surg* 1976; **42**: 182–8.
82. BROWN HM, GORLIN RJ. Oral mucosal involvement in nevus unius lateris (ichthyosis hystrix). A review of the literature and report of a case. *Arch Dermatol* 1960; **81**: 509–15.
83. BUCHNER A, HANSEN LS. Pigmented nevi of the oral mucosa: a clinicopathologic study of 32 new cases and review of 75 cases from the literature. Part I. *Oral Surg* 1979; **48**: 131–42.
84. BUCHNER A, HANSEN LS. Pigmented nevi of the oral mucosa: a clinicopathologic study of 32 new cases and review of 75 cases from the literature. Part II. Analysis of 107 cases. *Oral Surg* 1980; **49**: 55–62.
85. BUCHNER A, HANSEN LS. Melanotic macule of the oral mucosa. A clinicopathologic study of 105 cases. *Oral Surg* 1979; **48**: 244–9.
86. BUCHNER A, HANSEN LS. Amalgam pigmentation (amalgam tattoo) of the oral mucosa. *Oral Surg* 1980; **49**: 139–47.
87. BUDTZ-JØRGENSEN E. Oral mucosal lesions associated with the weaving of removable dentures. *J Oral Pathol* 1981; **10**: 65–80.
88. BUNNEY MH. Contact dermatitis in beekeepers due to propolis (beeglue). *Br J Dermatol* 1968; **80**: 17–23.
89. BURKETT LW. *Oral medicine. Diagnosis and treatment.* 6 ed. Philadelphia: JB Lippincott Co, 1972.
90. BURKITT DP. The discovery of Burkitt's lymphoma. *Cancer* 1983; **51**: 1777–86.
91. BUTLER DJ, THOMPSON H. Malignant granuloma. *Br J Oral Surg* 1972; **9**: 208–21.
92. CADY B, CATLIN D. Epidermoid carcinoma of the gum. A 20-year survey. *Cancer* 1969; **23**: 551–69.
93. CAHN LR. The denture sore mouth. *Ann Dent* 1936; **3**: 33–6.
94. CALHOUN NR, JOHNSON CC. Oral manifestations of mycosis fungoides. Report of a case. *Oral Surg* 1966; **22**: 261–4.
95. CAMPBELL CH. Pigmentation of the nail beds, palate and skin occurring during malarial suppressive therapy with "Camoquin". *Med J Aust* 1960; **47**: 956–8.
96. CARRERAS AL. Lesiones mucocutaneas producidas por Leishmania braziliensis. *Acta Odontol Venez* 1974; **12**: 3–21.
97. CASSINGHAM RJ. Infectious mononucleosis. A review of the literature, including recent findings on etiology. *Oral Surg* 1971; **31**: 601–23.
98. CATALDO E, BERKMAN MD. Cysts of the oral mucosa in newborns. *Am J Dis Child* 1968; **116**: 44–8.
99. CATALDO E, McCARTHY P, YAFFEE H. Psoriasis with oral manifestations. *Cutis* 1977; **20**: 705–8.
100. CAWSON RA. Chronic oral candidiasis and leukoplakia. *Oral Surg* 1966; **22**: 582–91.
101. CAWSON RA. Leukoplakia and oral cancer. *Proc R Soc Med* 1969; **62**: 610–15.
102. CAWSON RA. Infections of the oral mucous membranes. In: COHEN B, KRAMER IRH, eds. *Scientific foundations of dentistry.* London: William Heinemann Medical Books Ltd, 1976; 484–97.
103. CAWSON RA, McSWIGGAN DA. An outbreak of hand-foot-and-mouth disease in a dental hospital. *Oral Surg* 1969; **27**: 451–9.
104. CELIS A, LITTLE JW. Clinical study of hairy tongue in hospital patients. *J Oral Med* 1966; **21**: 139–45.
105. CERNÉA P, CRÉPY C, KUFFER R, MASCARO JM, BADILLET G, MARIE JL. Aspects peu connus des candidoses buccales. Les candidoses à foyers multiples de la cavité buccale. *Rev Stomatol* (Paris) 1965; **66**: 103–38.
106. CERNÉA P, KUFFER R, BROCHERIOU C. L'épithélioma sur lichen plan buccal. *Actual Odonto-Stomatol* 1971; No. 96: 473–90.
107. ČERVENKA J, GORLIN RJ, ANDERSON VE. The syndrome of pits of the lower lip and cleft palate and/or palate. Genetic considerations. *Am J Hum Genet* 1967; **19**: 416–32.
108. ČERVENKA J, SHAPIRO BL. Cleft uvula in Chippewa Indians: prevalence and genetics. *Hum Biol* 1970; **42**: 47–52.

320

109. CHANDRA K, RATNAKAR C, RAMACHANDRAN PC, PARKASH S. Rhinosporidiosis of the parotid duct. *J Laryngol Otol* 1971; **85**: 1083–5.
110. CHAUDHRY AP, VICKERS RA, GORLIN RJ. Intraoral minor salivary gland tumors. An analysis of 1,414 cases. *Oral Surg* 1961; **14**: 1194–1226.
111. CHAUDHRY AP, YAMANE GM, SHARLOCK SE, RAJ MS, JAIN R. A clinicopathological study of intraoral lymphoepithelial cysts. *J Oral Med* 1984; **39**: 79–84.
112. CHEN S-Y, FANTASIA JE, MILLER AS. Myxoid lipoma of oral soft tissue. *Oral Surg* 1984; **57**: 300–7.
113. CHOMETTE G, AURIOL M, TEREAU Y, VAILLANT JM. Les tumeurs mucoepidermoides des glandes salivaires accessoires. *Ann Pathol* 1982; **2**: 29–40.
114. CHORZELSKI TT, BENTNER EH, JABLONSKA S, BLASZCZYK M, TRIFTSHAUSER C. Immuno-fluorescence studies in the diagnosis of dermatitis herpetiformis and its differentiation from bullous pemphigoid. *J Invest Dermatol* 1971; **56**: 373–80.
115. CHUE PWY. Acute angioneurotic edema of the lips and tongue due to emotinal stress. *Oral Surg* 1976; **41**: 734–8.
116. CHUNG CP, NISENGARD RJ, SLOTS J, GENCO RJ. Bacterial IgG and IgM antibody titers in acute necrotizing ulcerative gingivitis. *J Periodontol* 1983; **54**: 557–62.
117. CLAUSEN FP. Histopathology of focal epithelial hyperplasia. Evidence of viral infection. *Dan Dent J* 1969; **73**: 1013–22.
118. COHEN L. Mucoceles of the oral cavity. *Oral Surg* 1965; **19**: 365–72.
119. COHEN WD, MORRIS AL. Periodontal manifestations of cyclic neutropenia. *J Periodontol* 1961; **32**: 159–68.
120. COHEN WD, SHAPIRO J, FRIEDMAN L, KYLE GC, FRANKLIN S. A longitudinal investigation of the periodontal changes during pregnancy and fifteen months postpartum: part II. *J Periodontol* 1971; **42**: 653–7.
121. COLBY RA, KERR DA, ROBINSON HBG. *Color atlas of oral pathology.* 3rd ed. Philadelphia: JB Lippincott Co, 1971.
122. COOKE BED. The diagnosis of bullous lesions affecting the oral mucosa. I. *Br Dent J* 1960; **109**: 83–96.
123. COOKE RA. Verrucous carcinoma of the oral mucosa in Papua-New Guinea. *Cancer* 1969; **24**: 397–402.
124. COUSTEAU C, LEYDER P, LAUFER J. Syphilis primaire buccale. Un diagnostic parfois difficile. *Rev Stomatol Chir Maxillofac* 1984; **85**: 391–8.
125. COWAN L. Gonococcal ulceration of the tongue in the gonococcal dermatitis syndrome. *Br J Vener Dis* 1969; **45**: 228–31.
126. CRAWFORD WH, KORCIIN L, GRESKOVICH FJ. Neurilemomas of the oral cavity. Report of five cases. *J Oral Surg* 1968; **26**: 651–8.
127. CROCKER AC. The histiocytosis syndrome. In: VAUGHAN VC, MCKAY RJ, eds. *Nelson textbook of paediatrics.* 10th ed. Philadelphia: Saunders, 1975; 1950–2.
128. CURTIS AB. Childhood leukemias; initial oral manifestations. *J Am Dent Assoc* 1971; **81**: 159–64.
129. DABELSTEEN E. Distribution of complement and immunoglobulin in oral pemphigus lesions. *Acta Dermatovenerol* 1978; **58**: 540–3.
130. DABELSTEEN E, ULLMAN S, THOMSEN K, RYGAARD J. Demonstration of basement membrane autoantibodies in patients with benign mucous membrane pemphigoid. *Acta Dermatovenerol* 1974; **54**: 189–92.
131. DAHLLÖF G, REINHOLT FP, HJERPE A, MODÉER T. A quantitative analysis of connective tissue components in the phenotoin-induced gingival overgrowth in children. *J Peridontal Res* 1984; **19**: 401–7.
132. DAMM DD, WHITE DK, BRINKER CM. Variations of palatal erythema secondary to fellatio. *Oral Surg* 1981; **52**: 417–21.
133. DANBOLT N. Acrodermatitis enteropathica. *Br J Dermatol* 1979; **100**: 37–40.
134. DANIELS TE. Labial salivary gland biopsy in Sjögren's syndrome. *Arthritis Rheum* 1984; **27**: 147–56.

135. DANIELSEN L. *Morphological changes in pseudoxanthoma elasticum and senile skin*. Thesis. *Acta Dermatovenerol* 1979, Suppl 83.

136. DANIELSEN L, KOBAYASHI T. Pseudoxanthoma elasticum: an ultrastructural study of oral lesions. *Acta Dermatovenerol* 1974; **54**: 173–6.

137. DAYAL PK, MANI NJ. Clinical aspects of the tongue in anemia. *Ann Dent* 1979; **38**: 21–6.

138. DEASY MJ, VOGEL RI, MACEDO-SOBRINKO B, GERTZMAN G, SIMON B. Familial benign chronic neutropenia associated with periodontal disease: a case report. *J Periodontol* 1980; **51**: 206–10.

139. DE JONG WFB, ALBRECHT M, BÁNÓCZY J, VAN DER WAAL I. Epithelial dysplasia in oral lichen planus. *Int J Oral Surg* 1984; **13**: 221–5.

140. DE-THÉ G, GESER A, DAY NE. Epidemiological evidence for causal relationship between Epstein-Barr virus and Burkitt's lymphoma from Ugandan prospective study. *Nature* 1978; **274**: 756–61.

141. DEVILDOS LR, LANGLOIS CC. Intramucosal cellular nevi. *Oral Surg* 1981; **52**: 162–6.

142. DONATSKY O. *Recurrent aphthous stomatitis. Immunological aspects*. Thesis. København 1978.

143. DORPH-PETERSEN L, PINDBORG JJ. Actinomycosis of the tongue. Report of a case. *Oral Surg* 1954; **7**: 1178–82.

144. DOUGLAS CW, GAMMON MD. Reassessing the epidemiology of lip cancer. *Oral Surg* 1984; **57**: 631–42.

145. DREIZEN S. Stomatotoxic manifestations of cancer chemotherapy. *J Prosthet Dent* 1978; **40**: 650–5.

146. DREIZEN S. MCCREDIE KB, KEATING MJ. Chemotherapy-associated oral hemorrhages in adults with acute leukemia. *Oral Surg* 1984; **57**: 494–8.

147. DREIZEN S, MCCREDIE KB, KEATING MJ, LUNA MA. Malignant gingival and skin "infiltrates" in adult leukemia. *Oral Surg* 1983; **55**: 572–8.

148. DUKES MNG. *Meyler's side effects of drugs. A survey of unwanted effects of drugs reported in 1972–1975*. Amsterdam: Excerpta Medica, 1975.

149. DUMMETT CO. Physiologic pigmentation of the oral and cutaneous tissues in the Negro. *J Dent Res* 1946; **25**: 421–32.

150. DUNNETT WN. Infectious mononucleosis. *Br Med J* 1963; **1**: 1187–91.

151. DWORKIN JP, HARTMAN DE. Progressive speech deterioration and dysphagia in amyotrophic lateral sclerosis: case report. *Arch Phys Med Rehabil* 1979; **60**: 423–5.

152. EASSON EC, PALMER MK. Prognostic factors in oral cancer. *Clin Oncol* 1976; **2**: 191–202.

153. EASTMAN JR, GOLDBLATT LI. Psoriasis. Palatal manifestations and physiologic considerations. *J Periodontol* 1983; **54**: 736–9.

154. EBBESEN P, BIGGAR RJ, MELBYE M, eds. *AIDS: a basic guide for clinicians*. Copenhagen: Munksgaard, 1984.

155. EBLING FJ, ROOK A. Disorders of keratinization. In: ROOK A, WILKINSON DS, EBLING FJG, eds. *Textbook of dermatology*. 3rd ed. Oxford: Blackwell Scientific Publications, 1979; 1294.

156. EDINGTON GM, GILLES HM. *Pathology in the tropics*. London: Edward Arnold Ltd, 1969.

157. EGELAND T, BRANDTZAEG P. Deposition of immunoglobulin and complement in muco cutaneous lesions related to treatment with D-penicillamine. *J Oral Pathol* 1982; **11**: 183–90.

158. EISENBERG E. Intraoral isolated herpes zoster. *Oral Surg* 1978; **45**: 214–9.

159. EISENBUD L, SCIUBBA J, MIR R, SACHS SA. Oral presentations in non-Hodgkins lymphoma: a review of thirty-one cases. Part I. Data analysis. *Oral Surg* 1983; **56**: 151–6.

160. EL-DIBANY MM, AZAB S, KUTTY MK. Breast carcinoma metastatic to the maxillary gingiva. *J Oral Maxillofac Surg* 1984; **42**: 459–61.

161. EL-GHOBAREY A et al. Dermatomyositis: observations on the use of immunosuppressive therapy and review of literature. *Postgrad Med J* 1978; **54**: 516–27.

162. ELLIS CN, VANDERVEEN EE, RASMUSSEN JE. Scurvy: a case caused by peculiar dietary habits. *Arch Dermatol* 1984; **120**: 1212–4.

163. EMSLIE RD. Cancrum oris. *Dent Practit Dent Rec* 1963; **13**: 481–95.

164. ENEROTH C-M. Incidence and prognosis of salivary gland tumours at different sites. A study of parotid, submandibular and palatal tumours in 2,632 patients. *Acta Otolaryngol* (Stockh) 1970; Suppl 263: 174–8.

165. ENEROTH C-M, HJERTMAN I, MOBERGER G. Adenoid cystic carcinoma of the palate. *Acta Otolaryngol* (Stockh) 1968; **66**: 248–60.

166. ENEROTH C-M, HJERTMAN L, MOBERGER G. Squamous cell carcinoma of the palate. *Acta Otolaryngol* (Stockh) 1972; **73**: 418–27.

167. ENWONWU CO. Infectious oral necrosis (cancrum oris) in Nigerian children: a review. *Community Dent Oral Epidemiol* 1985; **13**: in press.

168. ENZINGER FM, LATTES R, TORLONI H. *Histological typing of soft tissue tumours*. Geneva: World Health Organization, 1969.

169. ERDMANN H. Das Wattenrollenulkus. *Schweiz Monatsschr Zahnheilkd* 1964; **74**: 326–8.

170. ETTINGER RL, MANDERSON RD. A clinical study of sublingual varices. *Oral Surg* 1974; **38**: 540–5.

171. EVERSOLE LR, JACOBSEN PL, STONE CE. Oral and gingival changes in systemic sclerosis (scleroderma). *J Periodontol* 1984; **55**: 175–8.

172. EVERSOLE LR, LEIDER AS, ALEXANDER G. Intraoral and labial keratoacanthoma. *Oral Surg* 1982; **54**: 663–7.

173. EVERSOLE LR, RINGER M. The role of dental restorative metals in the pathogenesis of oral lichen planus. *Oral Surg* 1984; **57**: 383–7.

174. EYRE J, NALLY FF. Oral candidosis and carcinoma. *Br J Dermatol* 1971; **85**: 73–5.

175. FALCONER DT. Scurvy presenting with oral symptoms. A case report. *Br Dent J* 1979; **146**: 313–4.

176. FANTASIA JE, MILLER AS. Papillary cystadenoma lymphomatosum arising in minor salivary glands. *Oral Surg* 1981; **52**: 411–6.

177. FARMAN AG. Clinical and cytological features of the oral lesions caused by chicken-pox (varicella). *J Oral Med* 1976; **31**: 94–8.

178. FARMAN AG. Atrophic lesions of the tongue among diabetic outpatients: their incidence and regression. *J Oral Pathol* 1977; **6**: 396–400.

179. FARMAN AG, KATZ J, ELOFF J, CYWES S. Mandibulofacial aspects of the cervical cystic lymphangioma (cystic hygroma). *Br J Oral Surg* 1978–79; **16**: 125–34.

180. FARMAN AG, KY S. Oral leiomyosarcoma. Report of case and review of the literature pertaining to smooth-muscle tumors of the oral cavity. *Oral Surg* 1977; **43**: 402–9.

181. FARMAN AG, UYS PB. Oral Kaposi's sarcoma. *Oral Surg* 1975; **39**: 288–96.

182. FARMAN AG et al. Central papillary atrophy of the tongue and denture stomatitis. *J Prosthet Dent* 1978; **40**: 253–6.

183. FAUCI AS, HAYNES BF, KATZ P, WOLFF SM. Wegener's granulomatosis: prospective clinical and therapeutic experience with 85 patients for 21 years. *Ann Intern Med* 1983; **98**: 76–85.

184. FEWINGS JD, LANDER H, ANDERSON KF, HENNING FR, RADDEN BG, JEANES BJ. Disseminated histoplasmosis. *Aust Ann Med* 1970; **2**: 151–8.

185. FINNE K, GÖRANSON K, WINCKLER L. Oral lichen planus and contact allergy to mercury. *Int J Oral Surg* 1982; **11**: 236–9.

186. FIORE-DONNO G, SAMSON J. Dépistage du pemphigus vulgaire: rôle du médecin-dentiste. *Schweiz Monatsschr Zahnheilkd* 1979; **89**: 1121–32.

187. FISHER AA. Allergic contact stomatitis. *Cutis* 1975; **15**: 149–53.

188. FITZPATRICK PJ, TEPPERMAN BS. Carcinoma of the floor of the mouth. *J Can Assoc Radiol* 1982; **33**: 148–53.

189. FITZPATRICK TB, EISEN AZ, WOLFF K, FREEDBERG IM, AUSTAN KF. *Dermatology in general medicine*. 2nd ed. New York: McGraw Hill Book Company, 1979.

190. FIUMARA NJ, GRANDE DJ, GIUNTA JL. Papular secondary syphilis of the tongue. *Oral Surg* 1978; **45**: 540–2.

191. FIUMARA NJ, LESELL S. Manifestations of late congenital syphilis. An analysis of 271 patients. *Arch Dermatol* 1970; **102**: 78–83.

192. FIUMARA NJ, LESELL S. The stigmata of late congenital syphilis: an analysis of 100 patients. *Sexually Transmitted Dis* 1983; **10**: 126–9.

193. FLETCHER JP, CRABB HSM. Fibrosarcomatous epulis. Report of a case. *Oral Surg* 1961; **14**: 1091–8.

194. FLØTRA L, GJERMO P, RØLLA G, WÆRHAUG J. Side effects of chlorhexidine mouth washes. *Scand J Dent Res* 1971; **79**: 119–25.

195. FOGH-ANDERSEN P. Incidence of cleft lip and palate constant or increasing? *Acta Chir Scand* 1961; **122**: 106–11.

196. FORSSLUND G. The occurrence of subepithelial gingival blood vessels in patients with morbus caeruleus (tetralogy of Fallot). *Acta Odontol Scand* 1962; **20**: 301–6.

197. FOSTER ME, NALLY FF. Benign mucous membrane pemphigoid (cicatricial mucosal pemphigoid): a reconsideration. *Oral Surg* 1977; **44**: 697–705.

198. FRASER FC. Etiology of cleft lip and palate. In: GRABB WC, ROSENSTEIN SW, BZOCH KR, eds. *Cleft lip and palate*. Boston: Little, Brown and Co, 1971; 54–65.

199. FRAZELL EL, LUCAS JC. Cancer of the tongue. Report of the management of 1,554 patients. *Cancer* 1962; **15**: 1085–99.

200. FREEMAN C, BERG JW, CUTLER SJ. Occurrence and prognosis of extranodal lymphomas. *Cancer* 1972; **29**: 252–60.

201. FREGERT S, KOLLANDER M, POULSEN J. Allergic contact stomatitis from gold denture. *Contact Dermatitis* 1979; **5**: 63–4.

202. GAMBLE JW, DRISCOLL EJ. Oral manifestations of macroglobulinemia of Waldenström. *Oral Surg* 1960; **13**: 104–10.

203. GARDNER DG. Peripheral ameloblastoma: a study of 21 cases, including 5 reported as basal cell carcinoma of the gingiva. *Cancer* 1977; **39**: 1625–33.

204. GARDNER DG, DALEY TD. The use of the terms monomorphic adenoma, basal cell adenoma, and canalicular adenoma as applied to salivary gland tumors. *Oral Surg* 1983; **56**: 608–15.

205. GEBEL K, HORNSTEIN OP. Drug-induced oral erythema multiforme. Results of a long-term retrospective study. *Dermatologica* 1984; **168**: 35–40.

206. GHOSE LJ, BAGHDADY VS. Prevalence og geographic and plicated tongue in 6090 Iraqi schoolchildren. *Community Dent Oral Epidemiol* 1982; **10**: 214–6.

207. GIANSANTI JS, TILLERY DE, OLANSKY S. Oral mucosal pigmentation resulting from antimalarial therapy. *Oral Surg* 1971; **31**: 66–9.

208. GISLEN G, NILSSON KO, MATSSON L. Gingival inflammation in diabetic children related to degree of metabolic control. *Acta Odontol Scand* 1980; **38**: 241–6.

209. GLENERT U. Drug stomatitis due to gold therapy – a clinical and histologic study. *Oral Surg* 1984; **58**: 52–6.

210. GOH KT, DORAISINGHAM S, TAN JL, LIM GN, CHEW SE. An outbreak of hand, foot, and mouth disease in Singapore. *Bull World Health Organization* 1982; **60**: 965–9.

211. GOOD AE. Reiter's disease: modern concepts. *Cutis* 1979; **24**: 514–23.

212. GORDON NC, BROWN S, KHOSLA VM, HANSEN LS. Lead poisoning. A comprehensive review and report of a case. *Oral Surg* 1979; **47**: 500–512.

213. GORLIN RJ, GOLDMAN HM. *Thoma's oral pathology*. 6th ed. St. Louis: C. V. Mosby Co, 1970.

214. GORLIN RJ, PINDBORG JJ, COHEN MM JR. *Syndromes of the head and neck*. 2nd ed. New York: McGraw-Hill Book Company, 1976.

215. GORLIN RJ, SEDANO HO, VICKERS RA, ČERVENKA J. Multiple mucosal neuromas, phaeochromocytoma and medullary carcinoma of the thyroid – a syndrome. *Cancer* 1968; **22**: 293–9.

216. GORSKY M, SILVERMAN S JR, LOZADA F, KUSHNER J. Histiocytosis X: occurrence and oral involvement in six adolescent and adult patients. *Oral Surg* 1983; **55**: 24–8.

217. GOSMAN JR, MILLER GA. Intraoral junctional nevus: review of the literature and report of a case. *J Oral Surg* 1975; **33**: 275–81.

324

218. GOULD MSE, PICTON DCA. The gingival condition of congenitally cyanotic individuals. *Br Dent J* 1960; **109**: 96–100.

219. GREEN D. Scleroderma and its oral manifestations. Report of three cases of progressive systemic sclerosis (diffuse scleroderma). *Oral Surg* 1962; **15**: 1312–24.

220. GREENBERG MS. Clinical and histologic changes of the oral mucosa in pernicious anemia. *Oral Surg* 1981; **52**: 38–42.

221. GREENSPAN D, GREENSPAN JS, CONANT M, PETERSEN V, SILVERMAN S JR, DESOUZA Y DE. Oral "hairy" leucoplakia in male homosexuals: evidence of association with both papillomavirus and a herpes-group virus. *Lancet* 1984; **2**: 831–4.

222. GREER RO, GOLDMAN HM. Oral papillomas. Clinicopathologic evaluation and retrospective examination in 110 lesions. *Oral Surg* 1974; **38**: 435–40.

223. GREER RO, POULSON TC. Oral tissue alterations associated with the use of smokeless tobacco by teen-agers. Part I. Clinical findings. *Oral Surg* 1983; **56**: 275–84.

224. GREWE JM, MCCOMBIE F. Prevalence of cleft uvula in British Columbia. *Angle Orthodont* 1971; **41**: 336–9.

225. GRIFFIN JM, BACH DE, NESPECA JA, MARSHALL KJ. Noma: report of two cases. *Oral Surg* 1983; **56**: 605–7.

226. GUGGENHEIM I, ISMAIL YH. Oral ulcerations associated with indomethacin therapy: report of three cases. *J Am Dent Assoc* 1975; **90**: 632–4.

227. GUPTA PC, MEHTA FS, DAFTARY DK *et al.* Incidence rates of oral cancer and natural history of oral precancerous lesions in a 10-year follow-up study of Indian villagers. *Community Dent Oral Epidemiol* 1980; **8**: 287–333.

228. GUPTA PC, PINDBORG JJ, MEHTA FS. Comparison of carcinogenicity of betel quid with and without tobacco: an epidemiological review. *Ecol Dis* 1982; **1**: 213–9.

229. HAIDAR Z, LAM PKP. Leukoplakia and lichen planus. *Br Dent J* 1981; **151**; 374–6.

230. HAKALA PE. Dental and oral changes in congenital heart disease. *Suom Hammaslääk Toim* 1967; **63**: 284–324.

231. HANEKE E. *Zungen- und Mundschleimhautbrennen.* München: Carl Hanser Verlag, 1980.

232. HANSEN JDL. Herpes simplex stomatitis in children: its clinical picture and complications as seen in Cape Town. *S Afr Med J* 1961; **35**: 131–3.

233. HANSEN LS, BUCHNER A. Changing concepts of the junctional nevus and melanoma: review of the literature and report of case. *J Oral Surg* 1981; **39**: 961–5.

234. HANSEN LS, SILVERMAN S JR, DANIELS TE. The differential diagnosis of pyostomatitis and its relation to bowel disease. *Oral Surg* 1983; **55**: 363–73.

235. HARTMAN KS. Histiocytosis X: a review of 114 cases with oral involvement. *Oral Surg* 1980; **49**: 38–54.

236. HASLER JF. The role of immunofluorescence in the diagnosis of oral vesiculobullous disorders. *Oral Surg* 1972; **33**: 362–74.

237. HASSE CD, ZOUTENDAM GL, GOMBAS OF. Intraoral blue (Jadassohn-Tieche) nevus. *Oral Surg* 1978; **45**: 755–61.

238. HASSELL T, O'DONNELL J, PEARLMAN J, TESINI D, MURPHY T, BEST H. Phenytoin induced gingival overgrowth in institutionalized epileptics. *J Clin Periodontol* 1984; **11**: 242–53.

239. HATZIOTIS JC. Lipoma of the oral cavity. *Oral Surg* 1971; **31**: 511–24.

240. HATZIOTIS JC, ASPRIDES H. Neurilemoma (schwannoma) of the oral cavity. *Oral Surg* 1967; **24**: 510–26.

241. HAY KD, MULLER HK, READE PC. D-penicillamine-induced mucocutaneous lesions with features of pemphigus. *Oral Surg* 1978; **45**: 385–95.

242. HAY KD, READE PC. The use of an elimination diet in the treatment of recurrent aphthous ulceration of the oral cavity. *Oral Surg* 1984; **57**:: 504–7.

243. HEDIN CA. Smokers' melanosis: occurrence and localization in the attached gingiva. *Arch Dermatol* 1977; **113**: 1533–8.

244. HEDIN CA, LARSSON Å. Physiology and pathology of melanin pigmentation with special reference to the oral mucosa. *Swed Dent J* 1978; **2**: 113–29.

245. HEMANI DD, GUPTA AK, SHARMA KK, SHARMA SD. Leiomyoma of the palate. *J Laryngol Otol* 1983; **97**: 471–7.

246. HEWITT WL. The penicillins. A review of strategy and tactics. *J Am Med Assoc* 1963; **185**: 264–72.
247. HICKS ML, TEREZHALMY GT. Herpesvirus hominis Type 1: a summary of structure, composition, growth cycle, and cytopathogenic effects. *Oral Surg* 1979; **48**: 311–8.
248. HIDANO A *et al.* Natural history of nevus of Ota. *Arch Dermatol* 1967; **95**: 187–95.
249. HIETANEN J. Clinical and cytological features of oral pemphigus. *Acta Odontol Scand* 1982; **40**: 403–14.
250. HIETANEN J, SALO OP, KANERVA L, JUVAKOSKI T. Study of the oral mucosa in 200 consecutive patients with psoriasis. *Scand J Dent Res* 1984; **92**: 50–4.
251. HJORTH N, JERVØE P. Allergic contact stomatitis and dermatitis from flavour of toothpaste. (In Danish with English summary). *Dan Dent J* 1967; **71**: 937–42.
252. HJORTH N, KORR H. Hand-foot-mouth disease. Eine neue exanthemische Kinderkrankheit. *Hautarzt* 1966; **17**: 533–7.
253. HJØRTING-HANSEN E, BERTRAM U. Oral aspects of pernicious anaemia. *Br Dent J* 1968; **125**: 266–70.
254. HJØRTING-HANSEN E, HOLST E. Morsicatio mucosae oris and suctio mucosae oris. An analysis of oral mucosal changes due to biting and sucking habits. *Scand J Dent Res* 1970; **78**: 492–9.
255. HJØRTING-HANSEN E, SCHMIDT H. Ulcerated granuloma eosinophilicum diutinum of the tongue. *Acta Dermatovenerol* 1961; **41**: 235–9.
256. HOFER P-Å, BERGENHOLTZ A. Oral manifestations in Urbach-Wiethe disease (lipoglyco-proteinosis, lipoid proteinosis; hyalinosis cutis et mucosae). *Odontol Revy* 1975; **26**: 39–58.
257. HOLLAND-MOVITZ R, RIMPLER M, RUDOLPH P-O. Allergie gegenüber Gold in der Mundhöhle. *Dtsch Zahnärztl Z* 1980; **35**: 963–7.
258. HOLMSTRUP P, BESSERMANN M. Clinical therapeutic and pathogenic aspects of chronic oral multifocal candidiasis. *Oral Surg* 1984; **56**: 388–95.
259. HOLMSTRUP P, DABELSTEEN E. Changes in carbohydrate expression of lichen planus affected oral epithelial cell membranes. *J Invest Dermatol* 1979; **73**: 364–7.
260. HOLMSTRUP P, PINDBORG JJ. Erythroplakic lesions in relation to oral lichen planus. *Acta Dermatovenerol* 1979; **59**: Suppl 85: 77–84.
261. HOLST E. Remission of gingival hyperplasia in acute leukemia. *Dan Dent J* 1965; **69**: 698–703.
262. HONMA T, SAITO T, FUJIOKA Y. Intraepithelial atypical lymphocytes in oral lesions of Behçet's syndrome. *Arch Dermatol* 1981; **117**: 83–5.
263. HORNSTEIN OP. Melkersson-Rosenthal syndrome: A neuro-mucocutaneous disease of complex origin. *Curr Probl Dermatol* 1973; **5**: 117–56.
264. HORNSTEIN OP, ed. *Entzündliche und systemische Erkrankungen der Mundschleimhaut.* Stuttgart: Georg Thieme Verlag, 1974.
265. HOVINGA J, ROODVOETS AP, GAILLARD J. Some findings in patients with uraemic stomatitis. *J Max-Fac Surg* 1975; **3**: 125–7.
266. HUDSON CD, VICKERS RA. Clinicopathologic observations in prodromal herpes zoster of the fifth cranial nerve. *Oral Surg* 1971; **31**: 494–501.
267. HUME WJ. Geographic stomatitis: a critical review. *J Dent* 1975; **3**: 25–43.
268. ILDSTAD ST, BIGELOW ME, REMENSNYDER JP. Squamous cell carcinoma of the mobile tongue. *Am J Surg* 1983; **145**: 443–9.
269. INOVAY I, BÁNÓCZY J. The role of electrical potential differences in the etiology of chronic diseases of the oral mucosa. *J Dent Res* 1961; **40**: 884–90.
270. ISACSSON G, SHEAR M. Intraoral salivary gland tumors: a retrospective study of 201 cases. *J Oral Pathol* 1983; **12**: 57–62.
271. ISHIMARU Y, NAKANO S, YAMAOKA K., TAKAMI S. Outbreaks of hand, foot, and mouth disease by enterovirus 71. *Arch Dis Childh* 1980; **55**: 583–8.
272. ISRAELSON H, BINNIE WH, HURT WC. The hyperplastic gingivitis of Wegener's granulomatosis. *J Periodontol* 1981; **52**: 81–7.

326

273. IZUTSU KT, SCHUBERT MM, TRUELOVE EL *et al.* The predictive value of elevated labial saliva sodium concentration: its relation to labial gland pathology in bone marrow transplant recipients. *Hum Pathol* 1983; **14**: 29–35.
274. JACOBSON S, SHEAR M. Verrucous carcinoma of the mouth. *J Oral Pathol* 1972; **1**: 66–75.
275. JAKOBSEN J. Oral pigmentation in Greenlanders. A clinical study. *Dan Dent J* 1968; **72**: 1141–54.
276. JAMSKY RJ. Gonococcal tonsillitis. *Oral Surrg* 1977; **44**: 197–200.
277. JAMSKY RJ, CHRISTEN AG. Oral gonococcal infections. Report of two cases. *Oral Surg* 1982; **53**: 358–62.
278. JELLIFFE DB. *The assessment of the nutritional status of the community.* Geneva: World Health Organization, 1966.
279. JENKINS WMM, THOMAS HC, MASON DK. Oral infections with Candida albicans. *Scot Med J* 1973; **18**: 192–200.
280. JENNISON RF. Thrush in infancy. *Arch Dis Childh* 1977; **52**: 747–9.
281. JENSON AB, LANCASTER WD, HARTMANN D-P, SKAFFER EL. Frequency and distribution of papillomavirus structural antigens in verrucae, multiple papillomas, and condylomata of the oral cavity. *Am J Pathol* 1982; **107**: 2128.
282. JEPSEN A, WINTHER JE. Mycotic infection in oral leukoplakia. *Acta Odontol Scand* 1965; **23**: 239–56.
283. JIMENEZ ML, RAMOS J, GARRINGTON G, BAER PN. The familial occurrence of acute necrotizing gingivitis in children in Colombia, South America. *J Periodontol* 1969; **40**: 414–6.
284. JOHNSTON RB, NEWMAN SL. Chronic granulomatous disease. *Pediatric Clin No Am* 1977; **24**: 365–76.
285. JONES RF MCNAB. The Paterson-Brown Kelly syndrome: its relationship to iron deficiency and postcricoid carcinoma I–II. *J Laryngol* 1961; **75**: 529–61.
286. JONSSON R, HEYDEN G, WESTBERG NG, NYBERG G. Oral mucosal lesions in systemic lupus erythematosus – a clinical, histopathological and immunopathological study. *Arthritis Rheum:* in press.
287. JORGENSEN RJ, SHAPIRA SD, SALINAS CF, LEVIN LS. Intraoral findings and anomalies in neonates. *Pediatrics* 1982; **69**: 577–82.
288. JOSEPH EA, MARE H, IRVING WR. Oral South American blastomycosis in the United States of America. Report of a case. *Oral Surg* 1966; **21**: 732–7.
289. JOWTSCHEFF I. Berufliche Veränderungen und Schädigungen im Bereich der Mundhöhle bei Arbeitern der Glasindustrie. *Dtsch Stomatol* 1967; **17**: 442–7.
290. JUEL-JENSEN BE, MACCALLUM FO. *Herpes simplex, varicella and zoster. Clinical manifestations and treatment.* London: William Heinemann Medical Books Ltd, 1972.
291. JØLST O. Sex difference in denture-induced mucosal irritation hyperplasia. *Dan Dent J* 1963; **67**: 545–54.
292. KASHANI HG, MACKENZIE IC, KERBER PE. Cytology of linea alba using a filter imprint technique. *Clin Prev Dent* 1981; **2**: 21–4.
293. KASLICK RS, BRUSTEIN HC. Epidermolysis bullosa. Review of the literature and report of a case. *Oral Surg* 1961; **14**: 1315–30.
294. KATZ R. Acrokeratosis verruciformis. In: FITZPATRICK TB *et al. Dermatology in general medicine.* 2nd ed. New York: McGraw Hill Book Company, 1979.
295. KELLER AZ. Alcohol, tobacco and age factors in the relative frequency of cancer among males with and without liver cirrhosis. *Am J Epidemiol* 1977; **106**: 194–202.
296. KERR DA. Granuloma pyogenicum. *Oral Surg* 1951; **4**: 158–76.
297. KERR, DA, MCCLATCHEY KD, REGEZI JA. Idiopathic gingivostomatitis. Cheilitis, glossitis, gingivitis syndrome; atypical gingivostomatitis, plasma-cell gingivitis, plasmocytosis of gingiva. *Oral Surg* 1971; **32**: 402–23.
298. KHAIRI MRA, DEXTER RN, BURZYNSKI NJ, JOHNSTON CC. Mucosal neuroma, pheochromocytoma and medullary thyroid carcinoma: multiple endocrine neoplasia type 3. *Medicine* 1975; **54**: 89–112.

299. KILLEY HC, KAY LW. Hereditary haemorrhagic telangiectasia. *Br J Oral Surg* 1970; **7**: 161–7.

300. KINIRONS MJ. Increased salivary buffering in association with a low caries experience in children from cystic fibrosis. *J Dent Res* 1983; **62**: 815–7.

301. KLEINSASSER O, KLEIN HJ. Basalzellenadenome der Speicheldrüsen. *Arch Klin Exp Ohr Nas Kehlkopfheilkd* 1967; **189**: 302–16.

302. KLEISS E. Zur Genese der Glossitis rhombica mediana. *Arch Ohr Nas Kehlkopfheilkd* 1949; **155**: 490–502.

303. KLOSTERMANN GF. *Pigmentfleckenpolypose: Klinische, histologische und erbbiologische Studien am sogenannten Peutz-Syndrom.* Stuttgart: Georg Thieme Verlag, 1960.

304. KNAPP MJ. Pathology of oral tonsils. *Oral Surg* 1970; **29**: 295–304.

305. KOUSA M. Clinical observations on Reiter's disease with special reference to the non-venereal aetiology. *Acta Dermatovenerol* 1978; **58**: Suppl 81.

306. KRAMER IRH, EL-LABBAN N, LEE KW. The clinical features and risk of malignant transformation in sublingual keratosis. *Br Dent J* 1978; **144**: 171–80.

307. KRAUT RA, BUHLER JE. Heroin-induced thrombocytopenic purpura. *Oral Surg* 1978; **46**: 637–40.

308. KRAUT RA, BUHLER JE, LARUE JR, ACEVEDO A. Amyloidosis associated with multiple myeloma. *Oral Surg* 1977; **43**: 63–8.

309. KROESE WFS. Immunosuppressive drugs. In: DUKES MNG, ed. *Meyler's side effects of drugs.* Vol. VIII. Amsterdam: Excerpta Medica, 1977; 1000–19.

310. KRUTCHOFF DJ, CUTLER I, LASKOWSKI S. Oral lichen planus: the evidence regarding potential malignant transformation. *J Oral Pathol* 1978; **7**: 1–7.

311. KUFFER R. Syphilis buccale. Paris: Encyclopédie Médio-Chirurgicale, 1971; 22061, A10.

312. KUFFER R, BROCHERIOU C, CERNEA P. Exfoliatio areata linguae et mucosae oris. *Rev Stomatol* (Paris) 1971; **72**: 109–19.

313. KUFFER R, NOBLE JP. Stomatite de la D-pénicillamine. *Rev Stomatol* (Paris) 1973; **74**: 309–20.

314. KUFFER R, PUCHAULT P. Psoriasis pustuleux et athropatique avec atteinte de la muqueuse buccale. *Rev Stomatol* (Paris) 1973; **74**: 605–12.

315. KYLE RA, LINMAN JW. Gingivitis and chronic idiopathic neutropenia: report of two cases. *Mayo Clin Proc* 1970; **45**: 494–504.

316. KÖVESI G, BÁNÓCZY J. Follow-up studies in oral lichen planus. *Int J Oral Surg* 1973; **2**: 13–9.

317. LANGLAIS RP, BRICKER SL, COTTONE JA, BAKER BR. *Oral diagnosis, oral medicine and treatment planning.* Philadelphia: WB Saunders Company, 1984.

318. LARSEN VK, PINDBORG JJ. Mercury intoxications including oral manifestations. *Dan Dent J* 1979; **83**: 307–10.

319. LASKARIS GC, NICOLIS G, CAPETONAKIS JP. Mycosis fungoides with oral manifestations. *Oral Surg* 1978; **46**: 40–2.

320. LASKARIS GC, SKLAVOUNOU A, STRATIGOS J. Bullous pemphigoid, cicatricial pemphigoid, and pemphigus vulgaris. A comparative clinical survey of 278 cases. *Oral Surg* 1982; **54**: 656–62.

321. LAUTTAMUS A, KASANEN A, OKSALA E, TAMMISALO E. Oral manifestations in uremia. *Proc Finn Dent Soc* 1974; **70**: 59–66.

322. LEE YW, GISSER SD. Squamous cell carcinoma on the tongue in a nine year renal transplant survivor. *Cancer* 1978; **41**: 1–6.

323. LEHNER T. Fine structural findings in recurrent oral ulceration. *Br Dent J* 1966; **121**: 454–6.

324. LEHNER T. Oral candidosis. *Dent Pract Dent Rec* 1967; **17**: 209–16.

325. LEHNER T. Pathology of recurrent ulceration in Behçet's syndrome. *J Pathol* 1969; **97**: 481–94.

326. LEHNER T. Immunologic aspects of recurrent oral ulcers. *Oral Surg* 1972; **33**: 80–5.

327. LEVER WF. *Pemphigus and pemphigoid.* Springfield: Thomas, 1965.

328

328. LEVINE J, KRUTCHKOFF DJ, EISENBERG E. Monomorphic adenoma of minor salivary glands: a reappraisal and report of nine new cases. *J Oral Surg* 1981; **39**: 101–7.

329. LIGHTERMAN I, WATANABE Y, HIDAKA T. Leprosy of the oral cavity and adnexa. *Oral Surg* 1962; **15**: 1178–94.

330. LIND PO, HURLEN B, KOPPANG H.S. Electrogalvanically-induced contact allergy of the oral mucosa. Report of a case. *Int J Oral Surg* 1984; **13**: 339–45.

331. LINDENBAUM JE, DYCK PC VAN, ALLEN RG. Hand, foot and mouth disease associated with Coxsackie virus Group B. *Scand J Infect Dis* 1975; **7**: 161–3.

332. LINDQUIST C, TEPPO L. Epidemiological evaluation of sunlight as a risk factor of lip cancer. *Br J Cancer* 1978; **37**: 983–9.

333. LINDQUIST SF, HICKEY AJ, DRANE JB. Effect of oral hygiene on stomatitis in patients receiving cancer chemotherapy. *J Prosthet Dent* 1978; **40**: 312–4.

334. LITTNER M, DAYAN D, KAFFE I, et al. Acute streptococcal gingivostomatitis. Report of five cases and review of literature. *Oral Surg* 1982; **53**: 144–7.

335. LIVERSEDGE RL. Oral malignant melanoma. *Br J Oral Surg* 1975; **13**: 40–55.

336. LOCKHART PB. Gingival pigmentation as the sole presenting sign of chronic lead poisoning in a mentally retarded adult. *Oral Surg* 1981; **52**: 143–9.

337. LOVAS GL, WYSECKI GP, DALEY TD. The oral blue nervus: histogenetic implications of its ultrastructural features. *Oral Surg* 1983; **55**: 145–50.

338. LOWRY RE, TEMPERO RM, DAVIS LF. Epidermoid cyst of the floor of the mouth. *J Oral Surg* 1979; **37**: 271–3.

339. LOZADA F, SILVERMAN S. Erythema multiforme: clinical characteristics and natural history in fifty patients. *Oral Surg* 1978; **36**: 628–36.

340. LOZADA F, SILVERMAN S JR, MIGLIORATI CA, CONANT MA, VOLBERDING PA. Oral manifestations of tumor and opportunistic infections in the acquired immunodeficiency syndrome (AIDS): findings in 53 homosexual men with Kaposi's sarcoma. *Oral Surg* 1983; **56**: 491–4.

341. LUCAS RB. *Pathology of tumours of the oral tissues.* 4th ed. Edinburgh & London: Churchill Livingstone, 1984.

342. LUCY MF, READE PC, HAY KD. Lichen planus: a theory of pathogenesis. *Oral Surg* 1983; **56**: 521–6.

343. LYNCH DP, CRAGO CA, MARTINEZ MG. Necrotizing sialometaplasia: a review of the literature and report of two additional cases. *Oral Surg* 1979; **47**: 63–9.

344. LYNCH MA, SHIP II. Initial oral manifestations of leukemia. *J Am Dent Assoc* 1967; **75**: 932–40.

345. LØE H, SILNESS J. Periodontal disease in pregnancy. I. Prevalence and severity. *Acta Odontol Scand* 1963; **21**: 533–51.

346. LØE H, SCHIØTT CR. The effect of suppression of the oral microflora upon the development of dental plaque and gingivitis. In: MCHUGH WD, ed. *Dental plaque.* Edinburgh: Livingstone, 1970; 247–55.

347. MACFARLANE TW, HENARSKA SJ. The microbiology of angular cheilitis. *Br Dent J* 1976; **140**: 403–6.

348. MACINTYRE DR, BRIGGS JC. Primary oral malignant melanoma. *Int J Oral Surg* 1984; **13**: 160–5.

349. MANTHORPE R, FROST-LARSEN K, ISAGER H, PRAUSE JU. Sjögren's syndrome. A review with emphasis on immunological features. *Allergy* 1981; **36**: 139–53.

350. MARDER MZ, DEESEN KC. Transformation of oral lichen planus to squamous cell carcinoma: a literature review and report of case. *J Am Dent Assoc* 1982; **105**: 55–60.

351. MARKS R, CZATNY D. Geographic tongue: sensitivity to the environment. *Oral Surg* 1984; **58**: 155–9.

352. MARQUARD JV, RACEY GL. Combined medical and surgical management of intraoral condyloma acuminata. *J Oral Surg* 1981; **39**: 459–61.

353. MASER ED. Oral manifestations of pachyonychia congenita: a report of a case. *Oral Surg* 1977; **43**: 373–8.

329

354. MASHBERG A, MORRISSEY JB, GARFINKEL L. A study of the appearance of early asymptomatic oral squamous cell carcinoma. *Cancer* 1973; **32**: 1435–45.
355. MASON C, GRISIUS R, MCKEAN P. Stomatitis medicamentosa associated with gold therapy for rheumatoid arthrtitis. *U. S. Navy Med* 1978; **69**: 23–5.
356. MATHÉ G, RAPPAPORT H, O'CONNOR GT, TORLONI H. *Histological and cytological typing of neoplastic diseases of haematopoietic and lymphoid tissues.* Geneva: World Health Organization, 1976.
357. MATSUMOTO K. NAKAGAWA K, KKANEKO Z. The gingival hyperplasia resulting from diphenylhydantoin in children and adults. *Int J Clin Pharmacol* 1975; **12**: 369–71.
358. MATTHEWS JB, MASON GI. Oral granular cell myoblastoma: an immunohistochemical study. *J Oral Pathol* 1982; **11**: 343–52.
359. MCCARTHY FP. Pyostomatitis vegetans. Report of three cases. *Arch Dermatol Syphilol* 1949; **60**: 750–64.
360. MCCARTHY P, SHKLAR G. A syndrome of pyostomatitis vegetans and ulcerative colitis. *Arch Dermatol* 1963; **88**: 913–9.
361. MCCARTHY PL, SHKLAR G. *Diseases of the oral mucosa.* 2nd ed. Philadelphia: Lea & Febiger, 1980.
362. MCCOY JM, ECKERT EF. Sialoadenoma papilliferum. *J Oral Surg* 1980; **38**: 691–3.
363. MCDONALD JS, CRISSMAN JD, GLUCKMAN JL. Verrucous carcinoma of the oral cavity. *Head Neck Surg* 1982; **5**: 22–8.
364. MCENERY ET, GAINES FP. Tongue-tie in infants and children. *J Pediatr* 1941; **18**: 252–5.
365. MEDAHO RM, RULLI MA, MARTINELLI C. The etiopathogenesis of gingival cysts: a histological and histochemical study of three cases. *Oral Surg* 1973; **35**: 510–20.
366. MEHNERT H. Zur Kenntnis der Oslerschen Krankheit und ihrer Bedeutung für die Stomatologie. *Dtsch Zahnärztl Z* 1956; **11**: 948–52.
367. MEHTA FS, PINDBORG JJ, HAMNER JE, et al. *Report on investigations of oral cancer and precancerous conditions in Indian rural populations, 1966–1969.* Copenhagen: Munksgaard, 1971.
368. MERRITT HH. *A textbook of neurology.* 2nd ed. Philadelphia: Lea & Febiger, 1959.
369. MESKIN LH, GORLIN RJ, ISAACSON RJ. Abnormal morphology of the soft palate. I. The prevalence of cleft uvula. *Cleft Palate J* 1964; **1**: 342–6.
370. MESSMER E. Zur klinischen Begutachtung gewerblicher Bleivergiftungen. *Med Klin* 1954; **49**: 218–23.
371. MEYER I, ABBEY LM. The relationship of syphilis to primary carcinoma of the tongue. *Oral Surg* 1970; **30**: 678–81.
372. MEYER I, SHKLAR G. The oral manifestations of acquired syphilis. *Oral Surg* 1967; **23**: 45–57.
373. MEYLER L, ed. *Side effects of drugs.* Excerpta Medica: Amsterdam, 1966; vol. 5.
374. MICHAUD M, BACHNER RL, BIXLER D, KAFRAWY AH. Oral manifestation of acute leukemia in children. *J Am Dent Assoc* 1977; **95**: 1145–50.
375. MICHAUD M, BLANCHETTE G, TOMICH CF. Chronic ulceration of the hard palate: first clinical sign of undiagnosed pulmonary tuberculosis. *Oral Surg* 1984; **57**: 63–7.
376. MILLARD LG, BARKER DJ. Development of squamous cell carcinoma in chronic discoid lupus erythematosus. *Clin Exp Dermatol* 1978; **3**: 161–6.
377. MILLER AS, ETZAY RP. Verruciform xanthoma of the gingiva: report of six cases. *J Periodontol* 1973; **44**: 103–5.
378. MISHKIN DJ, AKERS JO, DARBY CP. Congenital neutropenia: report of a case a biorationale for dental management. *Oral Surg* 1976; **42**: 738–45.
379. MIYAKE H, TANAHA J. A new finding in oral cavity in pseudoxanthoma elasticum. *Nagoya J Med Sci* 1966; **19**: 251–9.
380. MORTENSEN H. Allergic stomatitis due to eugenol: report of a case. *Dan Dent J* 1968; **72**: 115–8.
381. MORTON RP, MISSOTHEN FEM, PHAROAH POD. Classifying cancer of the lip: an epidemiologic perspective. *Eur J Cancer Clin Oncol* 1983; **19**: 875–9.

330

382. Mosher DB, Fitzpatrick TB, Ortonne J-P. Abnormalities of pigmentation. In: Fitzpatrick TB *et al. Dermatology in general medicine.* 2nd ed. New York: McGraw Hill Book Company, 1979.

383. Moskow BS, Weinstein MM. Further observations on the gingival cyst: three case reports. *J Periodontol* 1975; **46**: 178–82.

384. Moskow BS, Bloom A. Embryogenesis of the gingival cyst. *J Clin Periodontol* 1983; **10**: 119–30.

385. Mostofi RS, Hayden NP, Soltani K. Oral malignant acanthosis nigricans. *Oral Surg* 1983; **56**: 372–4.

386. Muller DL, Silverberg SG, Penn I, Hammond WS. Squamous cell carcinoma of the skin and lip in renal homograft recipients. *Cancer* 1976; **37**: 729–34.

387. Murti PR, Bhonsle RB, Mehta FS, Daftary DK. Oro-facial lesions of tuberous sclerosis: a report on 7 cases. *Int J Oral Surg* 1980; **9**: 292–7.

388. Myllärniemi S, Perheentupa J. Oral findings in the autoimmune polyendocrinopathy-candidosis syndrome (CAPECS) and other forms of hypoparathyroidism. *Oral Surg* 1978; **45**: 721–9.

389. Najjar TA. Harmful effects of "aspirin compounds". *Oral Surg* 1977; **44**: 64–70.

390. Nasu M, Takagi M, Ishikawa G. Sialoadenoma papilliferum: report of a case. *J Oral Surg* 1981; **39**: 367–9.

391. Natiella JR, Neiders ME, Green GW. Oral leiomyoma. *J Oral Pathol* 1982; **11**: 353–65.

392. Neumann-Jensen B. Angioneurotic edema of the tongue. *Dan Dent J* 1978; **82**: 233–5.

393. Neumann-Jensen B, Holmstrup P, Pindborg JJ. Smoking habits of 611 patients with oral lichen planus. *Oral Surg* 19977; **43**: 410–5.

394. Newton AV. Denture sore mouth. *Br Dent J* 1962; **112**: 357–60.

395. Nilsen R, Livden J, Thunold S. Oral lesions of epidermolysis bullosa acquisita. *Oral Surg* 1978; **45**: 749–54.

396. Nishimura Y, Yakata H, Kawasaki T, Nakajima T. Metastatic tumours of the mouth and jaws. A review of the Japanese literature. *J Max-Fac Surg* 1982; **10**: 253–8.

397. Nizel AE. *The science of nutrition and its application in clinical dentistry.* 2nd ed. Philadelphia: WB Saunders Co.,1966.

398. Nordenram Å, Landt H. Hyperplasia of the oral tissues in denture cases. *Acta Odontol Scand* 1969; **27**: 481–91.

399. Nyquist G. A study of denture sore mouth. *Acta Odontol Scand* 1952; **10**: Suppl. 9.

400. O'Driscoll PM. Papillary hyperplasia of the palate. *Br Dent J* 1965; **118**: 77–80.

401. O'Duffy JD, Lehner T, Barmes CG. Summary of the Third International Conference on Behçet's Disease. *J Rheumatol* 1983; **10**: 154–8.

402. Oikarinen VJ, Calonius PEB, Sainio P. Metastatic tumours to the oral region. I. An analysis of cases in the literature. *Proc Finn Dent Soc* 1975; **71**: 58–65.

403. Oppenheim H, Livingston CS, Nixon JW, Miller CD. Streptomycin therapy in oral tuberculosis. *Arch Otolaryngol* 1950; **52**: 910–29.

404. Orban B. Discolorations of the oral mucous membrane by metallic foreign bodies. *J Periodontol* 1956; **17**: 55–65.

405. Örn G. Akzidentelle Vakzinestomatitis und Angina. *Acta Dermatovenerol* 1942; **23**: 35–45.

406. Overall JC. Oral herpes simplex: pathogenesis, clinical and virologic course, approach to treatment. In: Hooks J, Jordan G, eds. *Viral infections in oral medicine.* Amsterdam: Elsevier North Holland Inc., 1982.

407. Pass RF, Whitley RJ, Whelchel JD, Diethelm AG, Reynolds DW, Slford CA. Identification of patients with herpes simplex virus after renal transplantation. *J Infect Dis* 1979; **140**: 487–92.

408. Patrikiou A, Papanicolaou S, Stylogianni E, Sotiriadous S. Peripheral ameloblastoma. Case report and review of the literature. *Int J Oral Surg* 1983; **12**: 51–5.

409. Pedersen NG, Worsaae N. Gingivale forandringer hos en patient med hereditær trombasteni. *Dan Dent J* 1979; **83**: 119–22.

410. PENN I. Tumor incidence in human allograft recipients. *Transplant Proc* 1979; **11**: 1047–51.
411. PERL P, PERL T, GOLDBERG B. Hydatid cyst in the tongue. *Oral Surg* 1972; **33**: 579–81.
412. PERZIN KH, GULLANE P, CLAIRMONT AC. Adenoid cystic carcinomas arising in salivary glands. A correlation of histologic features and clinical course. *Cancer* 1978; **42**: 265–82.
413. PETERSEN J, HALBERG P, HØJGAARD K, LYON BB, ULLMAN S. Penicillamineinduced polymyositis-dermatomyositis. *Scand J Rheumatol* 1978; **7**: 113–7.
414. PFISTER H, HETTICH I, RUNNE V, GISSMANN L, CHIEF GN. Characterization of human papillomavirus type 13 from focal epithelial hyperplasia Heck lesions. *J Virol* 1983; **47**: 363–6.
415. PINDBORG JJ. Gingivitis in military personnel with special reference to ulcero-membranous gingivitis. *Odontol Tidskr* 1951; **59**: 405–99.
416. PINDBORG JJ. *Oral cancer and precancer.* Bristol: John Wright & Sons Ltd, 1980.
417. PINDBORG JJ, BARMES DE, ROED-PETERSEN B. Epidemiology and histology of oral leukoplakia and leukoedema among Papuans and New Guineans. *Cancer* 1968; **22**: 379–84.
418. PINDBORG JJ, BHAT M, DEVANATH KR, NARAYANA HR, RAMACHANDRA S. Occurrence of acute necrotizing gingivitis in South Indian children. *J Periodontol* 1966; **45**: 546–54.
419. PINDBORG JJ, BHAT M, ROED-PETERSEN B. Oral changes in severe protein deficiency in South Indian children with special reference to periodontal conditions. *J Periodontol* 1967; **38**: 218–21.
420. PINDBORG JJ, GORLIN RJ. Oral changes in acanthosis nigricans (juvenile type). Survey of the literature and report of a case. *Acta Dermatovenerol* 1962; **42**: 63–71.
421. PINDBORG JJ, GORLIN RJ, ASBOE-HANSEN G. Reiter's syndrome. Review of the literature and report of a case. *Oral Surg* 1963; **16**: 551–60.
422. PINDBORG JJ, HARDER F. Palatal necrotizing sialometaplasia. *Ugeskr Laeg* 1977; **139**: 657–9.
423. PINDBORG JJ, HILLERUP S. Carcinoma of the buccal mucosa in a 38-year renal transplant survivor. *Dan Dent J* 1984; **88**: 402–4.
424. PINDBORG JJ, KRAMER IRH, TORLONI H. *Histological typing of odontogenic tumours, jaw cysts, and allied lesions.* Geneva: World Health Organization, 1971.
425. PINDBORG JJ, MEHTA FS, DAFTARY DL, GUPTA PC, BHONSLE RB. Prevalence of oral lichen planus among 7,639 villagers in Kerala, South India. *Acta Dermatovenerol* 1972; **52**: 216–20.
426. PINDBORG JJ, MEHTA FS, GUPTA PC, DAFTARY DK, SMITH CJ. Reverse smoking in Andhra Pradesh, India: a study of palatal lesions among 10,169 villagers. *Br J Cancer* 1971; **25**: 10–20.
427. PINDBORG JJ, MURTI PR, BHONSLE RB, GUPTA PC, DAFTARY DK, MEHTA FS. Oral submucous fibrosis as a precancerous condition. *Scand J Dent Res* 1984; **92**: 224–9.
428. PINDBORG JJ, REIBEL J, ROED-PETERSEN B, MEHTA FS. Tobacco-induced changes in oral leukoplakic epithelium. *Cancer* 1980; **45**: 2330–6.
429. PINDBORG JJ, RENSTRUP G, POULSEN HE, SILVERMAN S JR. Studies in oral leukoplakias. V. Clinical and histologic signs of malignancy. *Acta Odontol Scand* 1963; **21**: 407–14.
430. PINDBORG JJ, ROED-PETERSEN B, RENSTRUP G. Role of smoking in floor of the mouth leukoplakias. *J Oral Pathol* 1972; **1**: 22–9.
431. PINDBORG JJ, SIRSAT SM. Oral submucous fibrosis. *Oral Surg* 1966; **22**: 764–79.
432. PINDBORG JJ, SØRENSEN NA. The condition of the oral mucosa and dentures in a Danish nursing home population. *Dan Dent J* 1983; **87**: 307–11.
433. PISANTI S, SHARAV Y, KAUFMAN E, POSNER LN. Pemphigus vulgaris: incidence in Jews of different ethnic groups according to age, sex, and initial lesion. *Oral Surg* 1974; **38**: 382–7.
434. PITTS W, PICKRELL K, QUINN G, MASSENGILL R. Electrical burns of lips and mouth in infants and children. *Plast Reconstr Surg* 1969; **44**: 471–9.
435. POGREL MA. Tumours of the salivary glands: a histological and clinical review. *Br J Oral Surg* 1979–80; **17**: 47–56.

332

436. POGREL MA, WELDON LL. Carcinoma arising in erosive lichen planus in the midline of the dorsum of the tongue. *Oral Surg* 1983; **55**: 62–6.
437. POLLOCK A. The leukemias. *Br Dent J* 1977; **142**: 369–72.
438. PRESCOTT LF. Antipyretic analgesics. In: DUKES MNG, ed. *Meyler's side effects of drugs.* Vol 8. Amsterdam: Excerpta Medica, 1977; 154–206.
439. PRÆTORIUS F, CLAUSEN PP. Immunohistochemical evidence of papilloma virus antigen in focal epithelial hyperplasia. *Dan Dent J* 1984; **89**: in press.
440. PRÆTORIUS-CLAUSEN F. Rare oral viral disorders. (Molluscum contagiosum, localized keratoacanthoma, verrucae, condyloma acuminatum and focal epithelial hyperplasia). *Oral Surg* 1972; **34**: 604–18.
441. PRÆTORIUS-CLAUSEN F, WILLIS JM. Papova virus-like particles in focal epithelial hyperplasia. *Scand J Dent Res* 1971; **79**: 362–5.
442. PUISSANT A, SCHIER J, KUFFER R, BADILLET G, SAURAT J-H. Histoplasmose disséminée. Traitement par le miconazole. *Ann Med Interne* 1978; **129**: 605–8.
443. RAHAMINOFF P, MUKSAM HV. Some observations on 1,246 cases of geographic tongue. *Am J Dis Child* 1957; **93**: 519–25.
444. RAHIMO AA, SHIMASAKI WW. Mercurial necrosis of the cheek. Report of a case. *Oral Surg* 1960; **13**: 54–8.
445. RAMASINGHE AW, WARNAKULASURIYA KAAS, TENNEKOON GE, SENEVIRATNA B. Oral mucosal changes in iron deficiency anemia in a Sri Lankan female population. *Oral Surg* 1983; **55**: 29–32.
446. RAPIDIS AD. Lipoma of the oral cavity. *Int J Oral Surg* 1982; **11**: 30–5.
447. RAPPAPORT I, SHIFFMAN MA. Multiple phlebectasia involving jejunum, oral cavity, and scrotum. *J Am Med Assoc* 1963; **185**: 437–40.
448. RASI HB, HERR BS, SPERER AV. Neurofibromatosis of the tongue. *Plast Reconstr Surg* 1965; **35**: 657–65.
449. RATEITSCHAK-PLÜSS EM, HEFTI A, LÖRTSCHER R, THIEL G. Initial observation that cyclosporin-A induces gingival enlargement in man. *J Clin Periodontol* 1983; **10**: 237–46.
450. RATZER ER, SCHWEITZER RJ, FRAZELL EL. Epidermoid carcinoma of the palate. *Am J Surg* 1970; **119**: 294–7.
451. REAUME CE, SOFIE VL. Lingual thyroid: review of the literature and report of a case. *Oral Surg* 1978; **45**: 841–5.
452. REDDY DG, RAO VK. Cancer of the palate in coastal Andhra due to smoking cigars with the burning end inside the mouth. *Indian J Med Sci* 1957; **11**: 791–8.
453. REDMAN RS, VANCE FL, GORLIN RJ, PEAGLER FD, MESKIN LH. Psychological component in the etiology of geographic tongue. *J Dent Res* 1966; **45**: 1403–8.
454. REES RT. Congenital ranula. *Br Dent J* 1979; **146**: 345–6.
455. REGEZI JA, DEEGAN MJ, HAYWARD JR. Lichen planus: immunologic and morphologic identification of the submucosal infiltrate. *Oral Surg* 1978; **46**: 44–52.
456. REGEZI JA, HAYWARD JR, PICKENS TN. Superficial malanomas of oral mucous membranes. *Oral Surg* 1978; **45**: 730–40.
457. REIBEL J, HARDER F. Intraoral adenolymphomas. *Dan Dent J* 1984; **88**: 564–8.
458. REICHART P. Pathologic changes in the soft palate in lepromatous leprosy. An evaluation of ten patients. *Oral Surg* 1974; **38**: 898–904.
459. REICHART P, DORNOW H. Gingivo-periodontal manifestation in chronic benign neutropenia. *J Clin Periodontal* 1978; **5**: 74–80.
460. RENNIE JS, MACDONALD DG, DAGG JH. Quantitative analysis of human buccal epithelium in iron deficiency anemia. *J Oral Pathol* 1982; **11**: 39–46.
461. RENSTRUP G, PINDBORG JJ. Salivary gland tumors in the palate. Report of 27 cases. *Acta Pathol Microbiol Scand* 1960; **49**: 417–25.
462. RICK G, HOWELL F, PINDBORG JJ. The peripheral ameloblastoma: a clinicopathologic study of 18 cases. 2nd Meeting of the International Association of Oral Pathologists, Noordwijkerhout, The Netherlands, 1984; Abstract.
463. RINTALA AE, RANTA R. Lower lip sinuses: 1. Epidemiology, microforms, and transverse sulci. *Br J Plast Surg* 1981; **34**: 25–30.

464. ROBINSON F. Lymphangioma of the tongue. *Br J Plast Surg* 1954; **6**: 48–56.
465. ROBINSON JE. Dental management of the oral effect of radiotherapy. *J Prosthet Dent* 1964; **14**: 582–7.
466. ROBINSON L, HUKILL PB. Hutchinson's melanotic freckle in oral mucous membrane. *Cancer* 1970; **26**: 297–302.
467. ROCKOFF AS. Chronic mucocutaneous candidiasis. *Arch Dermatol* 1979; **115**: 322–3.
468. RODU B, GOCKERMAN JP. Oral manifestations of the chronic graft-v-host reaction. *J Am Med Assoc* 1983; **249**: 504–7.
469. ROYER JE, HENDRICKSON DA, SCHARF HO. Phenytoin-induced hyperplasia of the pre-eruptive stage. *Oral Surg* 1983; **56**: 365–7.
470. ROED-PETERSEN B, RENSTRUP G. A topographical classification of the oral mucosa suitable for electronic data processing. Its application to 560 leukoplakias. *Acta Odontol Scand* 1969; **27**: 681–95.
471. ROLLER NW, GARFUNKEL A, NICHOLS C, SHIP II. Amyotrophic lateral sclerosis. *Oral Surg* 1974; **37**: 46–52.
472. ROOK A. Diseases of the lips. In: ROOK A, WILKINSON DS, EBLING FJG, eds. *Textbook of dermatology*. 3rd ed. Oxford: Blackwell Scientific Publications, 1979; 1903–8.
472a.ROYER JE, HENRICHSON DA, SCHARPF HO. Phenytoin-induced hyperplasia of the pre-eruptive stage. *Oral Surg* 1983; **56**: 365–7.
473. RUD J. Cervicofacial actinomycosis. *J Oral Surg* 1967; **25**: 229–35.
474. RUSHTON MA. Hereditary or idiopathic hyperplasia of the gums. *Dent Practit Dent Rec* 1957; **7**: 136–46.
475. SAMARANAYAKE LP, MACFARLANE TW. A retrospective study of patients with recurrent chronic atrophic candidosis. *Oral Surg* 1981; **52**: 150–3.
476. SANNER JR, RAMIN JE, YANG C-H. Carcinoma of the lung metastatic to the gingiva: review of the literature and report of case. *J Oral Surg* 1979; **37**: 103–6.
477. SAWYER DR, AROLE G, MOSADOMI A. Focal epithelial hyperplasia. Report of three cases from Nigeria, West Africa. *Oral Surg* 1983; **56**: 185–9.
478. SCHIFF L, ed. *Diseases of the liver*. 3rd ed. Philadelphia: JB Lippincott Co, 1969.
479. SCHIMPF A. Dermatitis herpetiformis (Duhring) zeitweise mit isoliertem Schleimhaut-befall. *Arch Klin Exp Dermatol* 1964; **220**: 250–60.
480. SCHIØDT M. Denture stomatitis with multiple intramucosal fistulae. *Scand J Dent Res* 1979; **87**: 50–7.
481. SCHIØDT M. Bivirkninger efter klorheksidinmundskylning. *Dan Dent J* 1980; **84**: 475–6.
482. SCHIØDT M. Oral manifestations of lupus erythematosus. Thesis. *Int J Oral Surg* 1984; **13**: 101–47.
483. SCHIØDT M, ANDERSEN L, SHEAR M, SMITH CJ. Leukoplakia-like lesions developing in oral discoud lupus erythematosus. *Acta Odontol Scand* 1981; **39**: 209–16.
484. SCHIØDT M, LARSEN V, BESSERMANN M. Oral findings in glassblowers. *Community Dent Oral Epidemiol* 1980; **8**: 195–200.
485. SCHIØDT M, PINDBORG JJ, KJÆRGAARD P. Burkitt's lymfom med kæbemanifestationer hos et dansk barn. *Dan Dent J* 1978; **82**: 402–7.
486. SCHIØDT M, WORSAAE N, HOLMSTRUP P, BAY L, ANDREASEN J, BESSERMANN M. Traumatic lesions of the gingiva provoked by toothbrushing. *Dan Dent J* 1979; **83**: 743–7.
487. SCHIØDT M, WORSAAE N, WADT J. Orale manifestationer ved Crohn's sygdom. *Dan Dent J* 1977; **81**: 426–9.
488. SCHLESINGER SL, BORBOTSINA J, O'NEILL L. Petechial hemorrhages of the soft palate secondary to fellatio. *Oral Surg* 1975; **40**: 376–8.
489. SCHMID U, HELBRON D, LENNERT K. Development of malignant lymphoma in myoepithe-lial sialadenitis (Sjögren's syndrome). *Virchows Arch (Pathol Anat)* 1982; **395**: 11–43.
490. SCHMIDT H, HJØRTING-HANSEN E, PHILIPSEN HP. Gonococcal stomatitis. *Acta Dermato-venerol* 1961; **41**: 324–7.
venerol 1961; **41**: 324–7.
491. SCHMITZ JF. A clinical study of inflammatory papillary hyperplasia. *J Prosthet Dent* 1964; **14**: 1034–9.

492. SCHNELL JD. Epidemiology and the prevention of peripartal mycoses. *Chemotherapy* 1982; **28** (Suppl 1): 66–72.

493. SCHUERMANN H. Glossitis und Pareiitis granulomatosa. Ein Beitrag zur "Cheilitis granulomatosa", Miescher bzw. zum "Melkersson-Rosenthal-Syndrom". *Hautarzt* 1952; **3**; 538–42.

494. SCHUERMANN H, GREITHER A, HORNSTEIN O. *Krankheiten der Mundschleimhaut und der Lippen.* 3. Aufl. München & Berlin: Urban & Schwarzenberg, 1966.

495. SCHUPPENER HJ. Das klinische Bild der Schleimhautbeteiligung bei Psoriasis pustulosa. *Arch Klin Exp Dermatol* 1960; **209**: 600–14.

496. SCHWARTZ RA. The keratoacanthoma: a review. *J Surg Oncol* 1979; **12**: 305–17.

497. SCOTT EP, STEIGMAN AJ. Accidental isolated primary vaccinia of the tongue. *J Pediatr* 1961; **58**: 77–9.

498. SCULLY C. Orofacial manifestations in tuberous sclerosis. *Oral Surg* 1977; **44**: 706–16.

499. SCULLY C, MACFADYEN E, CAMPBELL A. Oral manifestations in cyclic neutropenia. *Br J Oral Surg* 1982; **20**: 96–101.

500. SEIBERT JS, SHANNON CJ, JACOWAY JR. Treatment of recurrent condyloma acuminatum. *Oral Surg* 1969; **27**: 398–409.

501. SEIFERT G, BULL HG, DONATH K. Histologic subclassification of the cystadenolymphoma of the parotid gland. *Virchows Arch A* 1980; **388**: 13–38.

502. SEIFERT G, RIEB H, DONATH K. Klassifikation der Tumoren der kleinen Speicheldrüsen. Pathohistologische Analyse von 160 Tumoren. *Laryngol Rhinol Otol* 1980; **59**: 379–400.

503. SEWARD MH. Local disturbances attributed to eruption of the human primary dentition. *Br Dent J* 1971; **130**: 72–7.

504. SEWARD MH. Eruption cyst: an analysis of its clinical features. *J Oral Surg* 1973: **31**: 31–5.

505. SEWERIN I. A clinical and epidemiologic study of morsicatio buccarum/labiorum. *Scand J Dent Res* 1971; **79**: 73–80.

506. SEWERIN I. *The sebaceous glands in the vermilion border of the lips and in the oral mucosa of man.* Thesis. *Acta Odontol Scand* 1975; **33**: Suppl 68.

507. SHAFER WG. Verruciform xanthoma. *Oral Surg* 1971; **31**: 784–9.

508. SHAFER WG, HINE MK, LEVY BM. *A textbook of oral pathology.* 4th ed. Philadelphia. WB Saunders Co, 1983.

509. SHAFER WG, WALDRON CA. Erythroplakia of the oral cavity. *Cancer* 1975; **36**: 1021–8.

510. SHAPIRO L, JUHLIN EA. Eosinophilic ulcer of the tongue. Report of two cases and review of the literature. *Dermatologica* (Basel) 1970; **140**: 424–50.

511. SHEAR M. Erythroplakia of the mouth. *Int Dent J* 1972; **22**: 460–73.

512. SHEAR M, PINDBORG JJ. Verrucous hyperplasia of the oral mucosa. *Cancer* 1980; **46**: 1855–62.

513. SHEIL AGR. Cancer in allograft recipients in Australia and New Zealand. *Transplant Proc* 1977; **9**: 1133–6.

514. SHIAU Y-Y, KWAN H-W. Submucous fibrosis in Taiwan. *Oral Surg* 1979; **47**: 453–7.

515. SHIP II, MILLER MF, RAM C. A retrospective study of recurrent herpes labialis (RHL) in a professional population, 1958–1971. *Oral Surg* 1977; **44**: 723–30.

516. SHKLAR G. Lichen planus as an oral ulcerative disease. *Oral Surg* 1972; **33**: 376–88.

517. SHKLAR G, MCCARTHY PL. Oral lesions of mucous membrane pemphigoid. A study of 85 cases. *Arch Otolaryngol* 1971; **93**: 354–64.

518. SHKLAR G, MEYER I. Vascular tumors of the mouth and jaws. *Oral Surg* 1965; **19**: 335–58.

519. SILVERMANN S, BEUMER J. Primary herpetic gingivostomatitis of adult onset. *Oral Surg* 1973; **36**: 496–503.

519a.SILVERMANN S, GORSKY M, LOZADA F. Oral leukoplakia and malignant transformation. A follow-up study of 257 patients. *Cancer* 1984; **53**: 563–8.

520. SIMON GB, BERSON SD, YOUNG CN. Blastomycosis of the tongue. *S Afr Med J* 1977; **52**: 82–3.

521. SIMPSON HE. Lymphoid hyperplasia in foliate papillitis. *J Oral Surg* 1964; **22**: 209–14.
522. SIST TC. An exophytic soft tissue mass of the buccal mucosa. *J Oral Pathol* 1979; **8**: 266–71.
523. SKLAVOUNOU AD, LASKARIS G, ANGELOPOULOS AP. Serum immunoglobulins and complement (C′3) in oral lichen planus. *Oral Surg* 1983; **55**: 47–51.
524. SLAVIN RE, SANTOS GW. The graft versus host reaction in Man after bone marrow transplantation: pathology, pathogenesis, clinical features, and implications. *Clin Immunol Immunopathol* 1973; **1**: 472–98.
525. SLOMIANY BL, AONO M, MURTY VLN, SLOMIANY A, LEVINE MJ, TABAK LA. Lipid composition of submandibular saliva from normal and cystic fibrosis individuals. *J Dent Res* 1982; **61**: 1163–6.
526. SLOOTWEG PJ, MÜLLER H. Verrucous hyperplasia or verrucous carcinoma. *J Max-Fac Surg* 1983; **11**: 13–9.
527. SMITH I. Cancrum oris. *J Max-Fac Surg* 1979; **7**: 293–6.
528. SOMAN SC, SIRSAT MV. Primary malignant melanoma of the oral cavity in Indians. *Oral Surg* 1974; **38**: 426–34.
529. SOUTHMAN JC, COLLEY IT. Hand, foot and mouth disease. *Br Dent J* 1968; **125**: 298–301.
530. SPOUGE JD, TROTT JR, CHESKO G. Darier -White's disease: a cause of white lesions of the mucosa. *Oral Surg* 1966; **21**: 441–56.
531. STANBACK JS, PEAGLER FD. Primary amyloidosis. Review of the literature and report of a case. *Oral Surg* 1968; **26**: 774–81.
532. STARK RB, ed. *Cleft palate. A multidiscipline approach.* New York: Hoeber Medical Division, 1968.
533. STEFANSSON K, WOLLMANN RL. S-100 protein in granular cell tumors (granular cell myoblastomas). *Cancer* 1982; **49**: 1834–8.
534. STEINER GA. Successful treatment of acrodermatitis enteropathica with zinc sulfate. *Am J Hosp Pharm* 1978; **35**: 1535–8.
535. STEINER M, ALEXANDER WN. Primary syphilis of the gingiva. *Oral Surg* 1966; **21**: 530–5.
536. STEWART D, KERNOHAN DC. Self-inflicted gingival injuries: gingivitis artefacta, factitial gingivitis. *Dent Practit* 1972; **22**: 418–26.
537. STRAKOSCH EA, NELSON LM. Postrhagadic scars. *Arch Dermatol Syphilol* (Chic) 1941; **43**: 664–71.
538. STRASSBURG M, KNOLLE G. *Farbatlas der Mundschleimhauterkrankungen.* Berlin: Die Quintessenz, 1968.
539. STREMPEL H, KLEIN G, FRIEDERICH HC. Dyskératose congénitale. Essais thérapeutiques. *Ann Dermatol Venereol* 1983; **110**: 145–8.
540. STRIBLING J, WEITZNER S, SMITH GV. Kaposi's sarcoma in renal allograft recipients. *Cancer* 1978; **42**: 443–6.
541. SUGAR AW. The management of dental extractions in cases of thrombasthenia complicated by the development of isoantibodies to donor platelets. *Oral Surg* 1979; **48**: 116–9.
542. SUMMERS L, BOOTH DR. Intraoral condyloma acuminatum. *Oral Surg* 1974; **38**: 273–8.
543. SURINGA DWR, BANK LJ, ACKERMAN AB. Role of measles virus in skin lesions and Koplik's spots. *N Engl J Med* 1970; **283**: 1139–42.
544. SVENDSEN IB, ALBRECHTSEN B. The prevalence of dyskeratosis follicularis (Darier's disease) in Denmark. *Acta Dermatovenerol* 1959; **39**: 256–69.
545. SWAIN AF, UNSWORTH DJ. Anti-gliadin antibodies in dermatitis herpetiformis. *J R Soc Med* 1981; **74**: 458–9.
546. SWANSON AE, SPOUGE JD. Traumatic hyperplasia of the gingiva-alveolar fibrosis. *J Can Dent Assoc* 1981; **47**: 52–6.
547. SWENSON HM, REDISH CH, MANNE M. Agranulocytosis: two case reports. *J Periodontol* 1965; **36**: 466–70.
548. SØNDERGAARD-PETERSEN H. The Di Guglielmo syndrome: a study of 17 cases. *Acta Med Scand* 1975; **198**: 165–74.
549. TAHIRI. Un cas de kyste hydatique de la langue. *J Franç Otorhino-laryngol* 1965; **14**: 327–30.

336

550. TAKAGI M *et al.* Oral manifestations of acute promyelocytic leukemia. *J Oral Surg* 1978; **36**: 589–93.
551. TALLGREN A. Alveolar bone loss in denture wearers as related to facial morphology. *Acta Odontol Scand* 1970; **28**: 251–70.
552. TEMPEST MN. Cancrum oris. *Br J Surg* 1966; **53**: 949–69.
553. THACKRAY AC, LUCAS RB. *Tumors of the major salivary glands.* Atlas of Tumor Pathology Second Series Fasc 10. Washington: Armed Forces Institute of Pathology, 1974.
554. THACKRAY A, SOBIN L. *Histological typing of salivary gland tumours.* Geneva: World Health Organization, 1972.
555. TIILILÄ I. *Epulis gravidarum.* Thesis. *Suom Hammaslääk Toim* 1962; **58**: Suppl 1.
556. TILLMAN HT. Oral and systemic changes in acute adult scurvy. *Oral Surg* 1961; **14**: 877–81.
557. TIMOSCA G, GAVRILITA L. Le granulome périphérique à cellules géantes des maxillaires. Étude sur 173 cas. *Rev Stomatol* (Paris) 1976; **77**: 587–97.
558. TOMICH CE, SHAFER WG. Lymphoproliferative disease of the hard palate: a clinicopathologic entity. *Oral Surg* 1975; **39**: 754–68.
559. TORNES K, BANG G. Traumatic eosinophilic granuloma of the gingiva. *Oral Surg* 1974; **38**: 99–102.
560. TURBINER S, GIUNTA J, MALONEY PL. Orificial tuberculosis of the lip. *J Oral Surg* 1975; **33**: 443–7.
561. TURRELL AJW. Allergy to denture-base materials – fallacy or reality. *Br Dent J* 1966; **120**: 415–22.
562. TURRELL AJW. Angular cheilosis and dentures. *Br J Dermatol* 1967; **79**: 331–8.
563. TOUYZ LZG, HILLE JJ. A fruit-mouthwash chemical burn. *Oral Surg* 1984; **58**: 290–2.
564. TYGSTRUP I, HAASE E, FLENSBORG EW. The diagnostic value of lip biopsy in mucoviscoidosis. *Acta Paediatr Scand* 1969; **58**: 208–9.
565. TYLDESLEY WR. Tobacco chewing in English coal miners. A preliminary report. *Br J Oral Surg* 1971; **9**: 21–8.
566. TYLDESLEY WR. Exfoliative cheilitis. *Br J Oral Surg* 1973; **10**: 357–9.
567. TYLDESLEY WR. Oral lichen planus. *Br J Oral Surg* 1974; **11**: 187–206.
568. TYLDESLEY WR. *Atlas of oral medicine.* London: Peter Wolfe Publications, 1978.
569. ULLMANN K. Über seltene und neue Formen der Leukoplakia mucosae oris. *Wien Klin Wochenschr* 1932; **45**: 840–52.
570. ULMANSKY M. Primary amyloidosis of oral structures and pharynx. Report of a case. *Oral Surg* 1962; **15**: 800–7.
571. ULRICH KH. Zur Frage der Veränderungen im Mund-Kiefer-Bereich bei Akromegalie. *Dtsch Zahnärztl Z* 1962; **17**: 252–5.
572. URRMAN JD, LOWENSTEIN MB, ABELES M, WEINSTEIN A. Oral mucosal ulceration in systemic lupus erythematosus. *Arthritis Rheum* 1978; **21**: 58–61.
573. VANHALE HM, ROGERS RS, DOYLE JA, SCHROETER AL. Immunofluorescence microscopic studies of recurrent aphthous stomatitis. *Arch Dermatol* 1981; **117**: 779–81.
574. VAN MAARSSEVEEN ACMT, VAN DER WAAL I, STAM J, VELDHUIZEN RW, VAN DER KWAST WAM. Oral involvement in sarcoidosis. *Int J Oral Surg* 1982; **11**: 21–9.
575. VEGERS JWM, SNOW GB, VAN DER WALL I. Squamous cell carcinoma of the buccal mucosa. *Arch Otolaryngol* 1979; **105**: 192–5.
576. VICKERY IM, MIDDA M. Dental complications of cytotoxin therapy in Hodgkin's disease – a case report. *Br J Oral Surg* 1976; **13**: 282–8.
577. VOGEL C, KÖHLER I, LANCHART W, REICHART P. Cyclosporin-A-induzierte Mundschleimhautveränderungen. *Dtsch Zahn Mund Kieferheilkd* 1984; **8**: 168–71.
578. WAHLI PN. The epidemiology of oral and oropharyngeal cancer. *Bull World Health Org* 1968; **38**: 495–521.
579. WALDENSTRÖM J. Iron and epithelium. Some clinical observations. *Acta Med Scand* 1938; Suppl 90: 380–97.
580. WALDENSTRÖM J. Macroglobulinemia. *Advanc Metab Disord* 1965; **2**: 115–58.

581. WALDRON CA. Oral epithelial tumors. In: GORLIN RJ, GOLDMAN HM, eds. *Thoma's oral pathology*. 6th ed. St. Louis: CV Mosby Co, 1970; 801–60.
582. WALDRON CA, SHAFER WG. Leukoplakia revisited. A clinicopathologic study 3256 oral leukoplakias. *Cancer* 1975; **36**: 1386–92.
583. WANNENMACHER MF, FORCK G. Mundschleimhautveränderungen beim Sturge-Weber-Syndrom. *Dtsch Zahnärztl Z* 1970; **25**: 1030–5.
584. WANSCHER B. Contact dermatitis from propolis. *Br J Dermatol* 1976; **94**: 451–5.
585. WATERHOUSE J, MUIR C, SHANMUGARATNAM K et al. *Cancer incidence in five continents.* Vol IV. IARC Scientific Publications No. 42. Lyon: International Agency for Research on Cancer, 1982.
586. WEARY PE, WHEELER CE, LINGAMFELTER CS, CAWLEY EP. Localized accidental vaccinia. *Arch Dermatol* 1960; **82**: 804–11.
587. WEATHERS DR, GRIFFIN JW. Intraoral ulcerations of recurrent herpes simplex and recurrent aphthae: two distinct clinical entities. *J Am Dent Assoc* 1970; **81**: 81–7.
588. WELLS RS, HIGGS JM, MACDONALD A, VALDIMARSSON H, HOLT PJL. Familial chronic muco-cutaneous candidiasis. *J Med Genet* 1972; **9**: 302–10.
589. WESTERHOLM N. Pathological changes in the oral mucosa in connection with influenza asiatica. *Odontol Tidskr* 1961; **69**: 5–11.
590. WHEELER CE. Patogenesis of recurrent herpes simplex affections. *J Invest Dermatol* 1975; **65**: 341–6.
591. WHITE GE. Oral manifestations of leukemia in children. *Oral Surg* 1970; **29**: 420–7.
592. WHO COLLABORATION CENTRE FOR ORAL PRECANCEROUS LESIONS. Definition of leukoplakia and related lesions: an aid to studies on oral precancer. *Oral Surg* 1978; **46**: 518–39.
593. WIESENFELD D, FERGUSON MM, FORSYTH A, MACDONALD DG. Allergy to dental gold. *Oral Surg* 1984; **57**: 158–60.
594. WILLIAMS BD, LEHNER T. Immune complexes in Behçet's syndrome and recurrent oral ulceration. *Br Med J* 1977; **1**: 1387–9.
595. WILSON CWM. Food sensitivities, taste changes, aphthous ulcers and atopic symptoms in allergic disease. *Ann Allergy* 1980; **44**: 302–7.
596. WINN D, BLOT W, SHY CM, PICKLE LW, TOLEDO MA, TRAUMENI JF. Snuff dipping and oral cancer among women in the Southern United States. *N Eng J Med* 1981; **304**: 745–9.
597. WITKOP CJ, WHITE JG, SAUK JJ, KING RA. Clinical, histologic cytologic, and ultrastructural characteristics of the oral lesions from hereditary mucoepithelial dysplasia. *Oral Surg* 1978; **46**: 645–57.
598. WITTMANN A-L. Macroglossia in acromegaly and hypothyroidism. *Virchows Arch A Pathol Anat Histol* 1977; **373**: 353–60.
599. WOMER R, CLARK JE, WOOD P, SABIO H, KELLEY TE. Dyskeratosis congenita: two examples of this multisystem disorder. *Pediatrics* 1983; **71**: 603–9.
600. WORSAAE N, CHRISTENSEN KO, BONDESEN S, JARNUM S. Melkersson-Rosenthal syndrome and Crohn's disease. *Br J Oral Surg* 1980; **18**: 254–8.
601. WORSAAE N, PINDBORG JJ. Granulomatous gingival manifestations of Melkersson-Rosenthal syndrome. *Oral Surg* 1980; **49**: 131–8.
602. WORSAAE N, SCHWARTZ O, PINDBORG JJ. Follow-up study of 14 oral granular cell tumors. *Int J Oral Surg* 1979; **8**: 133–9.
603. WORSAAE N, WANSCHER B. Oral injury caused by fellatio. *Acta Dermatovenerol* 1978; **58**: 187–8.
604. WRIGHT BA. Median rhomboid glossitis: not a misnomer. *Oral Surg* 1978; **46**: 806–14.
605. WRIGHT BA, FENWICK F. Candidiasis and atrophic tongue lesions. *Oral Surg* 1981; **51**: 55–61.
606. WRIGHT JM, BALCINNAS BA, MUUS JH. Mycosis fungoides with oral manifestations. Report of a case and review of the literature. *Oral Surg* 1981; **51**: 24–31.
607. WRIGHT JM, DUNSWORTH AR. Follicular lymphoid hyperplasia of the hard palate: a benign lymphoproliferative process. *Oral Surg* 1983; **55**: 162–8.

608. WRIGHT JM, RANKIN KV, WILSON JW. Traumatic granuloma of the tongue. *Head Neck Surg* 1983; **5**: 363–6.
609. WRIGHT WE, DAVIS ML, GEFFEN DB, MARTIN SE, NELSON MJ, STRAUSS SE. Alveolar bone necrosis and tooth loss: a rare complication associated with herpes zoster infection of the fifth cranial nerve. *Oral Surg* 1983; **56**: 39–46.
610. WYK CW VAN. The oral lesion caused by aspirin: a clinicopathological study. *J Dent Assoc S Afr* 1967; **22**: 1–7.
610a.WYK CW VAN, AMBROSIO SC, VAN DER VYVER TC. Abnormal keratohyalin-like forms in leukoedema. *J Oral Pathol* 1984; **13**: 271–81.
611. WYK CW VAN, STAZ J, FARMAN AG. The chewing lesion of the cheeks and lips: its features and prevalence among a selected group of adolescents. *J Dent* 1977; **5**: 193–9.
612. WYNDER EL, BROSS IJ, FELDMAN RM. A study of the etiological factors in cancer of the mouth. *Cancer* 1957; **10**: 1300–23.
613. WYSOCKI GP, BROOKE RI. Oral manifestations of chronic grannulomatous disease. *Oral Surg* 1978; **46**: 815–9.
614. WYSOCKI GP, GRETZINGER HA, LAUPACIS A, ULAN RU, STILLER CR. Fibrous hyperplasia of the gingiva: a side effect of cyclosporing A therapy. *Oral Surg* 1983; **55**: 274–8.
615. YOUNG WG. Familial white folded dysplasia of the oral mucous membranes. *Br J Oral Surg* 1967; **5**: 93–8.
616. ZAHORSKY J. Herpangina. *Arch Pediatr* 1924; **41**: 181–4.
617. ZEGARELLI DJ, ZEGARELLI-SCHMIDT EC, ZEGARELLI EV. Verruciform xanthoma. *Oral Surg* 1975; **40**: 246–56.
618. ZEGARELLI DJ, ZEGARELLI EV. Intraoral pemphigus vulgaris. *Oral Surg* 1977; **44**: 384–93.
619. ZINSSER F. *Syphilis und syphilisähnliche Erkrankungen des Mundes.* Berlin: Urban & Schwarzenberg, 1912.

CODING OF CONTENT OF THE ATLAS ACCORDING TO:
INTERNATIONAL CLASSIFICATION OF DISEASES
APPLICATION TO DENTISTRY AND STOMATOLOGY
ICD-DA (1978)

I. INFECTIVE AND PARASITIC DISEASES

II. NEOPLASMS

* Refers to the numerical index of morphology of neoplasms (ICD–O).

X. DISEASES OF THE GENITOURINARY SYSTEM

XI. COMPLICATIONS OF PREGNANCY

XII. DISEASES OF THE SKIN AND SUBCUTANEOUS TISSUE

XIII. DISEASES OF THE MUSCULOSKELETAL SYSTEM AND CONNECTIVE TISSUE

XIV. CONGENITAL ANOMALIES

XVI. SYMPTOMS, SIGNS AND ILL-DEFINED CONDITIONS

XVII. INJURY AND POISONING

346

INDEX

(Page numbers in italics refer to the principal discussion of a subject)

347

INDEX
ACCORDING TO GEOGRAPHIC PATHOLOGY